Therapeutic Pediatric Nutrition

Let thy food be thy medicine and thy medicine be thy food

—Hippocrates

Therapeutic Pediatric Nutrition

Madhu Sharma
MSc Foods and Nutrition
Dietician
Department of Pediatrics
Advanced Pediatric Center
Postgraduate Institute of Medical Education
and Research (PGIMER), Chandigarh, India

Foreword
BNS Walia

JAYPEE BROTHERS MEDICAL PUBLISHERS (P) LTD
New Delhi • St Louis • Panama City • London

Published by
Jaypee Brothers Medical Publishers (P) Ltd

Corporate Office
4838/24 Ansari Road, Daryaganj, **New Delhi** - 110002, India
Phone: +91-11-43574357, Fax: +91-11-43574314

Offices in India

- **Ahmedabad**, e-mail: ahmedabad@jaypeebrothers.com
- **Bengaluru**, e-mail: bangalore@jaypeebrothers.com
- **Chennai**, e-mail: chennai@jaypeebrothers.com
- **Delhi**, e-mail: jaypee@jaypeebrothers.com
- **Hyderabad**, e-mail: hyderabad@jaypeebrothers.com
- **Kochi**, e-mail: kochi@jaypeebrothers.com
- **Kolkata**, e-mail: kolkata@jaypeebrothers.com
- **Lucknow**, e-mail: lucknow@jaypeebrothers.com
- **Mumbai**, e-mail: mumbai@jaypeebrothers.com
- **Nagpur**, e-mail: nagpur@jaypeebrothers.com

Overseas Offices

- **North America Office, USA,** Ph: 001-636-6279734
  e-mail: jaypee@jaypeebrothers.com, anjulav@jaypeebrothers.com
- **Central America Office, Panama City, Panama,** Ph: 001-507-317-0160,
  e-mail: cservice@jphmedical.com, Website: www.jphmedical.com
- **Europe Office, UK,** Ph: +44 (0) 2031708910, e-mail: info@jpmedpub.com

Therapeutic Pediatric Nutrition

First Edition: **2011**
ISBN 978-93-5025-262-8
Typeset at JPBMP typesetting unit
Printed at Rajkamal Electric Press, Plot No. 2, Phase-IV, Kundli, Haryana.

Dedicated to

The memory of my beloved late parents,
whose encouragement and aspirations inspired me
to achieve what I have today

Foreword

Diet and disease are intimately related. Diet modification and diet restriction has been practised since the birth of medicine. As our understanding of altered physiology of the body in disease state has improved with new research, dietetics has become a more and more scientific profession, rather than being just a catering and diet presentation service in a hospital setting (which unfortunately is still practised in some hospitals).

This book is a compendium of more than two decades of experience of Madhu Sharma in the pediatric section of a leading institution in India. The complex and serious clinical problems that enter the portals of this institution, require a coordinate effort by a multidisciplinary team of experts to restore a sick child to health and put him back to the path of normal health and development. In modern era, technical skill and recent advances in therapeutics often attract more attention, sometimes to the detriment of holistic medical care. It is often forgotten that care of a disease, does not necessarily ensure future health, which depends essentially upon good nutrition.

This book covers dietetic management of common as well as uncommon diseases of childhood. Each chapter is complete in itself and delineates in detail, every aspect of therapeutic dietetics, covering physiological background, pathogenesis of factors leading to nutritional disorders, nutritional requirements in the particular disease entity, the scientific basis of the menu planning and development of recipes, to provide the calculated amounts of nutrients in a palatable form.

Although every chapter follows the same scheme of presentation, the chapters on diabetes mellitus, kidney disorders, celiac disease and enteral feeing need special mention as examples of sound instructions. Rare disorders like inborn errors of metabolism are also covered. The nutritional aspects of a child in the intensive care are not neglected.

The rationale of every recommendation is firmly based on scientific data. Numerous tables in the text summarize the important recommendations, whereas the references reflects the extensive study based upon which the book is founded. The recipes display the experimental spirit of the author, who presents the selected dishes which are acceptable to children, are home-based and therefore affordable.

I consider the book to be a most comprehensive collection of current thoughts on therapeutic dietetics for the sick child. It should be on the shelf of every medical library, pediatricians, pediatric nurses and hospital dieticians. Every one of them will benefit from the insights of the experienced author on what to feed a sick child and how to offer it. The book will serve a great need in promoting early recovery and sustain growth of the sick child, especially those suffering from complex or chronic diseases.

BNS Walia
Emeritus Professor Pediatrics
Former Director
Postgraduate Institute of Medical Education and Research (PGIMER)
Chandigarh, India

Preface

He that takes medicine and neglects diet, wastes the skill of a physician
—Chinese Proverb

In my earlier book *Basic Pediatric Nutrition*, I had dealt with issues of feeding a normal, disease-free child and ways of maintaining a healthy diet pattern. But, there is also another angle to nutritional issues of children that being the type of nutrition required for the sick child.

Often, it is observed that children during illness lose appetite and are unable to eat optimally. However, their requirements actually increase during illness due to the catabolic state that they are in, and hence, providing the right diet to the child becomes a great challenge. Besides, there are a number of diseases encountered among children, where dietary restrictions are required, e.g. in malabsorptive conditions like celiac disease, cystic fibrosis or even inflammatory bowel disease. Treatment of celiac disease comprises only dietary modifications and so it is the case of cystic fibrosis. Constipation in children is one of the most common problems encountered by pediatricians and dieticians. In fact, it could be a consequence of faulty diet pattern itself, which requires appropriate dietary counseling of the parents or caregivers.

There are an increasing number of children presenting with Type II diabetes of childhood. As with adults, along with insulin, management is based on what and how much a child should eat. In fact, most often, the dose of insulin also needs to be based on the dietary intake of the child. This is where the role of medical nutrition therapy comes in. There is another very common entity prevalent in children, that of seizures or epilepsy as it is largely known. In cases of uncontrolled seizures, it is a type of specifically calculated and designed diet regimen—the ketogenic diet which is known to control such seizures effectively.

Information regarding therapeutic dietary regimens for children is available in a number of books as part of larger chapters or along with those applicable to adults. In this book, an attempt has been made to deal with diseases related specifically to the pediatric population and discuss all common as well as not so common diseases in a single compilation. Besides, care has been taken to deal with the therapeutic aspects in a simple and easily comprehensible format.

I hope this book shall be of great help to all students of Nutrition and Dietetics, as also nurses and clinicians associated with some nutritional care of a pediatric population. It would also serve as a useful guide for all trainers involved in the teaching of nutrition in colleges and other health care institutions.

Madhu Sharma

Acknowledgments

I wholeheartedly acknowledge the inspiration received by Dr Walia to continue my effort to bring out a sequel to my first book on *Basic Pediatric Nutrition* for the benefit of all those closely associated with pediatric nutrition. His valuable suggestions from time to time during the writing of the manuscript have helped me shape my small endeavor to give shape to this compilation. I also thank all my friends and colleagues for their constant support and encouragement to complete this book. The help provided by my student Saloni in organizing the manuscript in the soft copy is highly appreciated.

Contents

Chapter 1 Protein Energy Malnutrition

The health and well-being of any individual is based on a combination of various factors. Besides diet and good nutrition, a host of contributory factors go a long way in preventing disease and malnutrition. These may be environmental, sociodemographic, immunization programs, provision of clean water supply and even psychosocial.

Environmental factors include parental education, socioeconomic status, living standards and child rearing practices.

Sociodemographic factors include breastfeeding practices, diet during illness for mother and child, maternal malnutrition, low birth weight babies, recurrent infections, etc.

According to WHO definition, malnutrition involves a cellular imbalance between supply of nutrients and energy and the body's demand for them to ensure normal growth, maintenance and specific tissue functions. Malnutrition accounts for more than 50 percent of all infant mortality in developing countries, especially in the below 5 year's age group.

The most common form of malnutrition in children is protein energy malnutrition (PEM), which earlier was also called protein calorie malnutrition (PCM). It has also been defined as a pathological state characterized by inadequate intake of proteins and calories in varying degrees commonly associated with infections.[1] Children between 6-36 months old are generally at high risk of falling prey to this condition, since they are more vulnerable to infections, especially gastrointestinal and measles. Death rates are high among children with untreated PEM, and the risk of dying increase with severity of the condition. Electrolyte imbalance, hypothermia and complicating infections are some of the causes of mortality in these children.

Causes of PEM: PEM occurs primarily due to food deprivation, but other factors play a major role also. These can be discussed as:

- ***Low birth weight and infections:*** Recurrent diarrhea, acute respiratory infections, other preventable infections like measles, tuberculosis, whooping cough and helminthes, can aggravate and complicate a pre-existing condition of low birth weight. Again maternal malnutrition is an important cause of low birth weight.

- ***Food deprivation:*** Poverty is one important cause of food deprivation in small children. Large families contribute to this problem and the priority of food distribution generally is for the male child followed by other male members in the family.
- ***Food taboos and myths:*** Even where resources are not a limiting factor, very often self-imposed restrictions regarding intake of food, can affect provision of adequate nutrients to the child. Food fads and myths related to consumption of specific type of foods at different phases of pregnancy or lactation and subsequently weaning practices can be a sole cause of food deprivation. Very often these fads and myths are interlinked with various cultural beliefs and/or religious beliefs. A common observation made is pertaining to infant feeding practices, where, in most rural classes colostrums is discarded as it is considered poisonous for the baby. The maternal diet is also restricted keeping in mind 'hot' or 'cold' foods which may be 'unsuitable for the infant. All such practices can go a long way to adversely affect the availability of essential macro and micronutrients required for adequate growth and development of the child.
- ***Ignorance:*** Many rural and urban mothers are quite ignorant of their infant's need for adequate nutrition. It's a common belief that milk is the 'best and only' food for a child, even after he has crossed the first 6 months of his life. They continue to breastfeed exclusively, well up to 12-24 months, making little effort to offer cereal supplements. Alternatively, if breast milk is inadequate, they will continue to feed diluted milk without introducing cereals. Even during illness of the child, solid food is withheld and the baby is kept on undiluted milk or tea with an occasional biscuit or so. Cereal, pulse base foods are considered 'heavy' for the child's liver. These factors further contribute to inadequate nutrient intake and subsequently growth failure.

PATHOGENESIS OF PEM

Gopalan in 1968 introduced a new hypothesis, that of 'adaptation'.[2] This was termed as 'dysadaptation', stating that kwashiorkor in fact was a failure of adaptation. This was explained on biochemical and hormonal factors. The malnourished child adapts himself to the unfavorable circumstances and to the calorie and protein gap. They reduce their activity, curtail their growth thereby bringing down the basal metabolic rate (BMR) and thus save energy for survival. This reduction in BMR and lack of insulating fat leads to hypothermia which may prove fatal.[2]

The basic adaptation to explain the mechanism was that the gradual wasting of muscle and subcutaneous fat would also protect certain other metabolic processes. Like, the essential amino acids are made available, which it was assumed, would enable the liver to maintain the synthesis of components essential for homeostasis, like serum albumin and β-lipoprotein. This could explain the absence of edema or fatty liver in marasmus.[3]

The high level of catabolic hormones including cortisol causes muscle and fat breakdown. The anabolic hormones like insulin and insulin like growth factors maintain near normal anabolism to prevent edema and fatty liver by enabling the synthesis of albumin and β-lipoproteins from the available pool of amino acids.

Another theory postulated in the pathogenesis of PEM is that of free radicals which are assumed to play a role in edema, skin changes and fatty liver. The free oxygen radicals which are toxic to cell membranes are produced during infections. In the malnourished child, deficiency of nutrients like vitamins A, C and E and selenium which are antioxidants can result in the accumulation of toxic free oxygen radicals. These further damage the liver cells resulting in kwashiorkor.

CLASSIFICATION OF PEM

Various parameters are used to classify PEM like, weight for age, height for age or weight for height. The most widely used accepted criterion is the weight for age. This has been done by various workers of different times. The most widely used are the Gomez classification and the Indian Academy of Pediatrics (IAP) classification.[4,5] as given in Tables 1.1 and 1.2.

Other classifications used are by Jellife in 1965 and Wellcome in 1970 (Tables 1.3 and 1.4)

Jelliffe's Classification: Proposed in 1965, it has been categorized into 4 classes as shown in Table 1.3.[6]

Wellcome Trust or International Classification: This is based on clinical assessment as suggested by Wellcome Trust in 1970. Besides weight for age, it also considers presence or absence of edema as seen in Table 1.4.[7]

SPECTRUM OF PEM

There are three forms of PEM recognized, based on the clinical presentations:

Table 1.1: The Gomez classification

% Expected	*Classification*	*Category of Nutritional Status Wt. for age*
>90%	Normal	Normal
76-90	Mild malnutrition	1st degree malnutrition
61-75	Moderate malnutrition	2nd degree malnutrition
< 60	Severe malnutrition	3rd degree malnutrition

Table 1.2: The IAP classification

% of Expected Weight (Wt. for age)	*Nutritional Classification**
>80%	Normal
71-80	Grade 1
61-70	Grade 2
51-50	Grade 3 (severe malnutrition)
<50	Grade 4 (severe malnutrition)

*If coexisting edema of nutritional origin, the letter K is suffixed along with grade of malnutrition to denote kwashiorkor

Table 1.3: Jelliffe's classification of PEM

Nutritional Status (PEM)	*Wt. for age (Harvard) % of expected*
Normal	>90
First degree	80-90
Second degree	70-80
Third degree	60-70
Fourth degree	<60

Table 1.4: Wellcome Trust classification

Weight for age (Boston) % of expected	*Edema*	*Clinical type of PEM*
60-80	+	Kwashiorkor
60-80	–	Underweight
<60	–	Marasmus
<60	+	Marasmic Kwashiorkor

- Kwashiorkor
- Marasmus
- Marasmic Kwashiorkor

  A picture of the various features of PEM can be had from Table 1.5

Kwashiorkor

The word 'kwashiorkor' was first described by Dr. Cicely Williams in 1933. The word originates from the African language- *Ga* of Ghana,

Table 1.5: Clinical features of PEM

Spectrum	*Clinical symptoms*	
	Always present	*Sometimes present*
Marasmus	Wasting	Hunger, Wizened appearance
Kwashiorkor	Edema	Mental changes: irritability, poor appetite Skin Changes: flaky paint dermatosis Hair: sparse, loose, straight
Marasmic Kwashiorkor	Wasting + Edema	Any of the above symptoms and signs

meaning the 'red boy' due to the characteristic pigmentation. Other workers from the West Indies described this as 'sugar baby' due to the characteristic 'prominent cheeks' and edema. This deficiency is known to occur with the coming of the second sib, when the child is displaced from the breast by another child. This condition is seen mostly in children in their second year of life, following abrupt weaning. They appear to be apathetic, irritable, weak and inactive, with the presence of edema and fatty liver. The edema is detected by the production of a definite pit on exerting moderate pressure for 3 seconds with the thumb over the lower end of the tibia and dorsum of the foot.

Initially, parents may miss these features and on the contrary be satisfied by the false image of a 'fatty child' But what is not generally realized by the lay person is that this fat appears typically on the belly and is commonly referred to as 'pot belly', but from his buttocks would be flat and give a wasted appearance (Figs 1.1A and B).

The typical signs of PEM are described by the following associated abnormalities:

- *Body:* All body parts, especially buttocks, arms and legs have decreased subcutaneous fat layer.
- *Skin:* The skin appears dry and flaky (flaky paint dermatosis). Hyperpigmented plaques may be visible over areas of trauma.
- *Hair*: It becomes thin, sparse and brittle. It also turns dull brown or red, giving an appearance of a 'flag sign'.
- *Nails:* There will be fissures or ridges and increased fragility.
- *Abdomen*: The presence of edema due to accumulation of ascetic fluid and also hepatomegaly (fatty liver), makes the abdomen appear distended.
- *Mouth:* Signs of vitamin B group deficiency-cheilosis, angular stomatitis and papillary atrophy are commonly present.
- *Behavior:* The child neither appears irritable and avoids social interaction, nor responds socially. They have a poor appetite and refuse to eat.

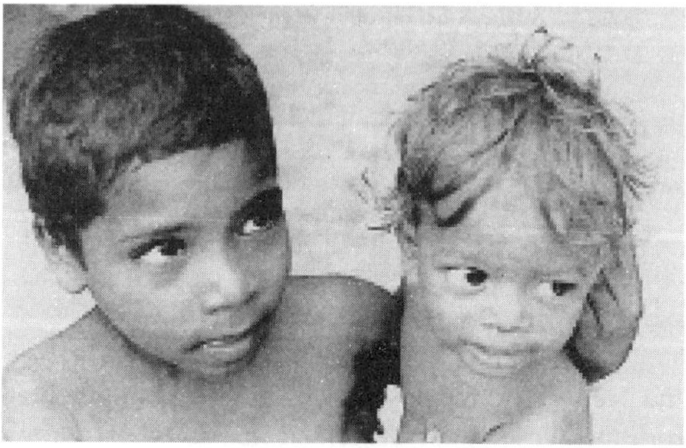

Fig. 1.1A: Child with sparse hair

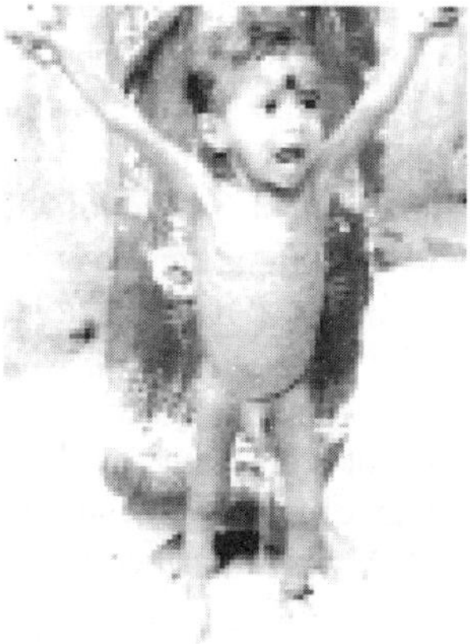

Fig. 1.1B: Child with pot belly

- *Deficiencies:* It is common to observe deficiency signs of vitamins, like, vitamin A, D and B group and minerals like iron and iodine.

MARASMUS

The term marasmus is derived from the Greek 'marasmos' which means wasting. In this condition, there is gross wasting of muscle and sub cutaneous tissues, marked stunting but no edema. This picture can be seen in early infancy unlike in kwashiorkor (Fig.1.2).

The marasmic condition is typical of sequel to prolonged starvation, chronic or recurrent infections and limited food intake. Marasmus represents an *adaptive* response to starvation, unlike kwashiorkor which

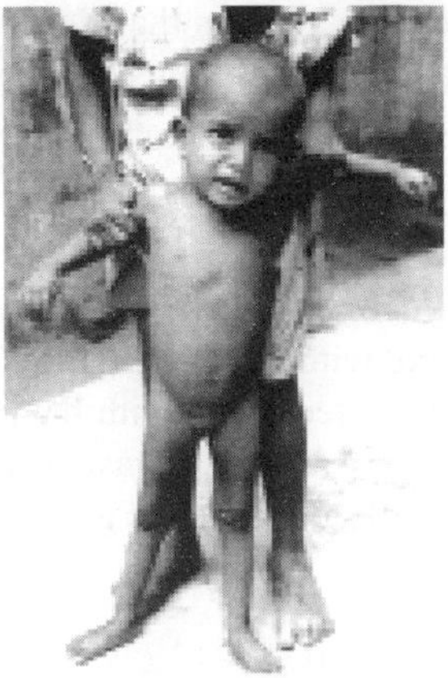

Fig. 1.2: Marasmic child

represents *maladaptive* response to starvation. In marasmus, the body utilizes all fat stores before using muscles. It is commonly seen in the first year of life due to lack of breastfeeding and the use of diluted animal milk. Poverty or famine like conditions and presence of diarrhea besides ignorance and poor maternal nutrition, are the precipitating factors. There is severe wasting of the shoulders, arms, buttocks and thighs with no visible rib outlines. The typical appearance of a marasmic child is described as:

- A 'thin old' man.
- Baggy pants (the loose skin of the buttocks hanging down)
- Child may be alert despite his condition.
- Absence of edema on the lower extremities.
- Prominent ribs.
- Large head with sunken eyes.
- A hungry child.
- Associated diarrhea or dehydration

In marasmus there is a marked deficit of weight but not as much in height. The marasmic infant has a good appetite but may also appear irritable, fretful and apathetic as in cases of kwashiorkor. Though the skin might appear dry, the typical characteristic peeling or patchy hypopigmentation may not be there.

It is worth mentioning here that during the past decade or so, the profile of PEM presenting in our hospitals has gradually changed. Frank cases of kwashiorkor are rarely encountered, but the marasmic type of picture is frequently observed. The prevalence of clinical form of malnutrition has been reduced to less than 1 percent. Hospital statistics also show that in recent years, admissions due to severe PEM have come down significantly.[8]

MARASMIC KWASHIORKOR

This condition is intermediary between marasmus and kwashiorkor, since such children present with a mixed picture. The body weight is less than 60 percent of the expected along with the presence of edema. The degree of stunting seems greater in marasmic kwashiorkor, indicating that duration of illness in this condition is greater than in kwashiorkor.

MANAGEMENT OF PEM

Treatment of severe malnutrition is a challenging task and involves multipronged approach. Most of the cases of severe malnutrition are not without complications on presentation. Severe infection is one major complication to be tackled. Management of these children involves hospitalization in majority of the cases. Noncomplicated cases can be managed on outpatient basis in a hospital or any primary health care center. But children presenting with complications can be managed in a hospital setting alone. Initial approach involves treating the complications first which may be:

Resuscitation

This involves tackling the life threatening medical emergencies on priority, which may include:

a. *Hypothermia/Hypoglycemia*: These are generally found together. The child is managed by keeping him warm and 'bedding in' with the mother is encouraged. Feeding if possible may be initiated. For hypoglycemia, the child is put on IV glucose10 percent, if immediate feeding is not possible. Child is treated for sepsis.
b. *Infections*: Infections are a major cause of mortality in PEM. Appropriate antibiotic therapy is initiated.
c. *Anemia*: If not managed appropriately, severe anemia may lead to heart failure. If required blood transfusion is resorted to.

Dehydration/Electrolyte Imbalance

Most often such children present with diarrhea. Depending upon the severity of stooling, ORS should be initiated. In moderate dehydration 70-100 ml/Kg ORS in 4 hours is given by sips. In severe dehydration, 100 ml/Kg normal saline or ringer lactate is given over 3-6 hours.

Mostly hypokalemia is present which can be managed by potassium supplement.

Congestive Heart Failure

In case of presence of heart failure, fluid intake is restricted and kept on maintenance dose. Diuretics may be given to prevent fluid overload.

Vitamin Deficiencies

Deficiency of vitamins is a common feature among children with PEM. Vitamin A can be supplemented in all cases. Vitamin K also is given to those with florid PEM and accompanied by diarrhea. All B complex vitamins, vitamin C, E and D too are administered along with calcium and zinc. Magnesium also needs to be supplemented if seizures, tetany or apathy are present.

Dietary Management

Different workers have laid down special formulae for achieving high energy intakes and to fulfill protein requirements for maximum catch-up growth rates.

The general pattern followed by them was of providing first class protein, in the form of milk protein powder, oil for energy along with sugar for flavor as well as extra energy. Oil is used to increase the density of the feed without increasing the bulk. Medium chain triglycerides are more desirable to enhance absorption and metabolism.

Almost all workers advocated regimens providing calories of around 150-200 per kg/d for maximum catch up growth. The protein requirements have been suggested around 3-4 g/Kg/d. But certain workers preferred to maintain calories at around 100 cal/kg/d initially and gradually increased over a week till the full volume is tolerated. This is specially so in children with kwashiorkor until the edema disappeared.

WHO in 1999,[9] laid down guidelines for routine treatment of severe malnutrition where the nutrition component was also stressed as follows:

Stabilization Phase—Initiate Refeeding

Feeding should be initiated gradually as soon as possible after admission. It should be formulated to provide just sufficient calories and proteins to maintain basic physiological functions. The main features include:

- Small frequent feeds of low osmalarity (<350) mOsm/L and low lactose (<2-3g/Kg/d)
- Oral or nasogastric feeds

- 100 cal./Kg/d-(not to exceed in initial phase)
- 1.0-1.5 g prot./Kg/d
- 130 ml/Kg/d of liquid (may begin with 100 ml/Kg/d if edema present)
- Feed should be of low viscosity, easy to prepare and socially acceptable.
- Continue breastfeeding if already doing so.

The above regimen is achieved using the F75 formula which is designed to provide 75 cals./100 ml and 0.9 g protein per 100 ml of the feed (Table 1.6). These should be fed by cup and spoon. The recommended schedule suggested is as shown in Table 1.7.

For children with good appetite, without edema, the schedule can be completed in 2-3 days. Careful monitoring should be done for:

- Amounts offered and left over
- Vomiting
- Stool frequency and consistency
- Daily body weight.

There may be accompanying diarrhea in some children, in which case milk based feeds can be replaced with soya based or any lactose free feeds till such time the stools settle down. Gradually low lactose feeds like curd may be initiated, and if tolerated, the amounts increased, and even milk based cereal feeds can be initiated.

In both types of PEM, basal energy expenditure increases gradually during refeeding. As the child loses weight, total body water as percentage of body weight increases and the child becomes relatively over hydrated. In children with edema, initiation of nutritional recovery is characterized by a progressive loss of extracellular fluid resulting in an initial loss of weight, followed by stabilization for 10-12 days and again followed by weight gain.[10]

Methods of feeding should be ideally from a cup and spoon along with continuation of breastfeeds. Even when breastfeeds are inadequate, non nutritive sucking should be encouraged which itself can enhance lactation. In case oral feeds are difficult to achieve, tubefeeding can be resorted to for a few days till such time oral feeding is restored adequately.

A weight gain of 0.5 Kg/week in children and 70 gms/week in infants is the goal. With recurrent infections this goal may be difficult; therefore control of infections is very important.

Catch-up Growth

This is the rehabilitation phase, when the appetite of the child is restored within 8-10 days, return of social smile and the child begins to take

Table 1.6: Recipes and composition of Starter formulae and catch-up formula

Ingredients	*Starter formula (F75)*	*Starter formula with cereal (F75)*	*Catch-up formula (F100)*
Dried skim milk (g)	25	25	80
Sugar (g)	100	70	50
Cereal flour (g)	-	35	-
Vegetable oil (ml)	27	27	60
Electrolyte mineral solution (ml)	20	20	20
Water: to make up to final soln. (ml)	1000	1000	1000
Contents per 100 ml			
Calories (kcal)	75	75	100
Protein (g)	0.9	1.1	2.9
Lactose (g)	1.3	1.3	4.2
Potassium (mmol)	4.0	4.2	6.3
Sodium (mmol)	0.6	0.6	1.9
Magnesium (mmol)	0.43	0.46	0.73
Zinc (mg)	2.0	2.0	2.3
Copper (mg)	0.25	0.25	0.25
Percent energy from protein	5	6	12
Percent energy from fat	32	32	53
Osmolality (mOsm/l)	413	334	419

(WHO, 2000).

Table 1.7: Feeding schedule for children with severe malnutrition

Days	*Froquency (hrly)*	*Vol./Kg/feed (ml)*	*Vol./Kg/d (ml)*
1–2	2	11	130
3–5	3	16	130
6–7+	4	22	130

interest in the surroundings. These are the first signs of recovery in a child with PEM. The increase in the feeds should be done gradually at this point to avoid risk of heart failure. To achieve the catch up growth the transition made is as follows:

- Replace F75 by F100 which contains 100 cal. and 2.9 g protein per 100 ml. This can be achieved by incorporating oil and sugar with milk or using milk cereal based preparations.
- Subsequently, the feeds are increased by 10-20 ml and finally 25-30 ml/Kg/feed. This can provide up till 200 cal./Kg/d.

- Monitoring for respiration and pulse rates are done regularly. The volume of feeds needs to be decreased as also the frequency (4 hourly) in case increase in respiration is observed. Once stabilized:
- Increased amounts of F100 formula at least 3-4 hourly can be started
- Calories given—150-200 kg/d
- Proteins increased—4-6 g/kg/d
- Continue breastfeeding
- Ensure administration of 6 monthly vitamin A dose.

The Indian Academy of Pediatrics in 2006 formed a working committee to bring out a revised consensus on the management of severely malnourished children in the Indian context,[11] which were adapted from the WHO guidelines of 2000 mentioned earlier. These guidelines are based on the hospital management of such children.

The modified formulae recommended for F75 and the catch-up formula F100 are as given in Tables 1.8 and 1.9 respectively.

Table 1.8: Starter diets F75

Diet contents (per 100 ml)	*F75 starter*	*F75 cereal based-(1)*	*F75 Cereal based-(2)*
Cow's milk (ml)	30	30	25
Sugar (g)	9	6	3
Cereal puffed rice (g)	-	2.5	6
Veget. Oil (ml)	2	2.5	3
Water- to make up to 100 ml	100	100	100
Calories (Kcal)	75	75	75
Proteins (g)	0.9	1.1	1.2
Lactose (g)	1.2	1.2	1.2

- Egg white can be replaced by 3 g of chicken or commercially available casein.
- Powdered puffed rice can be replaced by commercial rice or precooked rice (in same amounts)

Table 1.9: Catch-up diets F100

Diets contents (per 100 mL)	*F100 catch-up*	*F-100 catch-up (cereal based) Example 1*
Cow's milk/toned dairy milk (ml)	95	75
Sugar (g)	5	2.5
Cereal: Puffed rice (g)	–	7
Vegetable oil (g)	2	2
Water to make (mL)	101	100
Energy (kcal)	100	100
Protein (g)	2.9	2.9
Lactose (g)	3.8	3

Source: IAP, 2006.[11]

Table 1.10: Starter lactose free diet

Egg white *(g)	5
Glucose (g)	3.5
Cereal flour: Powdered puffed rice** (g)	7
Vegetable oil (g)	4
Water to make (mL)	100
Energy (kcal)	75
Protein (g)	1
Lactose	-

*Egg white may be replaced by 3 g of chicken or commercially available pure protein like casein.
**Powdered puffed rice may be replaced by commercial precooked rice preparations (in same amounts).
(*Source:* IAP, 2006).

Table 1.11: Catch-up lactose free diet

Egg white *(g)	20
Glucose or sugar (g)	4
Cereal Flour: Puffed rice** (g)	12
Vegetable oil (g)	4
Water to make (mL)	100
Energy (kcal)	100
Protein (g)	3
Lactose (g)	–

*Egg white may be replaced by 3 g of chicken or commercially available pure protein like casein.
**Powdered puffed rice may be replaced by commercial precooked rice preparations (in same amounts).
(*Source:* IAP, 2006).

The cereal-based low lactose (lower osmolarity) diets are recommended as starter diets for those with persistent diarrhea.[12] Lactose free diets are rarely needed for persistent diarrhea as most children do well on the above-mentioned, low lactose F75 diets. Children with persistent diarrhea, who continue to have diarrhea on the low lactose diets, should be given lactose (milk) free starter diets, as shown in Table 1.10.[13]. They can be followed on to lactose free catch-up diets as shown in Table 1.11

The low lactose catch up diets F100, can be started at the rehabilitation phase as shown in Table 1.12.

Complementary foods should be added as soon as possible to prepare the child for home foods at discharge. They should have comparable energy and protein concentrations once the catch-up diets are well tolerated. Khichri, dalia, banana, curd-rice and other culturally acceptable and locally available diets can also be offered liberally.

Table 1.12: Low lactose catch-up diets (F100)

Catch-up low lactose diets	*Example 1*	*Example 2*
Milk (cow's milk or toned dairy milk)	25 ml	25 ml
Egg white *(g)	12	–
Roasted powdered groundnut	–	5 g
Vegetable oil (g)	4	
Cereal flour: Powdered puffed rice** (g)	12	12
Energy (kcal)	100	100
Protein (g)	2.9	2.9
Lactose (g)	1	1

*Egg white may be replaced by 3 g of chicken or commercially available pure protein like casein.
**Powdered puffed rice may be replaced by commercial precooked rice preparations (in same amounts). Jaggery could be used instead of glucose/sugar.
(*Source:* IAP, 2006).

Nutrition recovery syndrome is a condition encountered generally during the rehabilitation phase of a child with severe PEM. It is marked by heptomegaly, gynacomastia, abdominal distension, ascites, splenomegaly, etc. This is attributed to sudden increase in energy and protein intake by these children. It is mostly self-limiting and might also be associated with tremors (kwashi shake) during treatment. Protein restriction during this period was generally advocated. But recently it has also been thought to result of excess hormones secreted during recovery phase.[14]

REFERENCES

1. WHO/FAO Expert Committee (1973), WHO Tech. Rep. Ser. No. 522.
2. Gopalan C. 1968. In: Calorie deficiencies and protein deficiencies pg. 49 (R.A. Mc Cance and E.M. Widdowson, Editors. Edinburgh and London: Churchill. Livingtone.
3. Alleyne G A O, Hay RW, Picou D I, Stanfield J.P. Brothers, New Delhi
4. Gomez F Ramos, Galvin R, et al. Mortality in second and third degree malnutrition. J Trop Prdiatr 1956;2:77-83.
5. Nutrition Sub Committee of the Indian Academy of Pediatrics, Report. Ind Pediatr. 1971;17:98-104.
6. Jelliffe D. B. (1966) WHO Monog Ser. No. 53.
7. Wellcome Trust Working party (1970). Lancet(ii0, 302.
8. Vinodini Reddy, In: Textbook of Human Nutrtition, (Ed). Mahtab S, Bamji N, Prahalad Rao, Vinodini Reddy 1996;252.
9. WHO. Management of the child with a serious infection or severe malnutrition. Guidelines for the care at the first referral level in developing countries; Geneva: WHO, 2000.

10. Fernando E. Viteri. Protein Energy Malnutrition; In: Textbook of Pediatric Nutrition, (Ed). Suskind RM, New York, Raven Press 1981;189-213.
11. Bhatnagar S, Lodha R, Chowdhary P, Sachdeva HPS, et al. IAP guidelines 2006 on hospital based management of severely malnourished children (Adapted from WHO guidelines) Ind Pediatr 2007;44:443-61.
12. Bhatnagar S, Bhan MK, Singh KD, Saxena SK, Shariff M. Efficiency of milk based diets in persistent diarrhea: A randomized controlled trial. Pediatrics 1996;98:1122-26.
13. Bhan MK, Bhandari N, Bhal R. Management of the severely malnourished child: Perspective from developing countries. BMJ 2003;326: 146-51.
14. Elizabeth KE. Protein energy malnutrition. In: Nutrition and Child Development, 3rd Ed. Paras Medical Publishers, 2004;133-7.

Chapter 2 Dietary Modification in Childhood Obesity

At one time the term childhood obesity was rarely seen in our country. The main nutritional problems in children focused around malnutrition which was in the form of undernutrtion, anemia and vitamin A deficiency. However, gradually, over a period of a decade or two, the other aspect of malnutrition, that of over nutrition in the form of childhood obesity has emerged as a major health problem in India too. In the USA childhood obesity has increased at least by 50 percent since 1976. It is well known that 80 percent of obese adolescents become obese adults. Overweight in adolescence predicts a broad range of adverse health affects that are independent of adult weight after 55 years of follow-up.[1]

Effective treatment and prevention of obesity must begin in childhood. However, studies indicate that care providers recommend initiation of treatment for only less than 20 percent of obese children.

The causes of higher rates of fatness in developing countries are poorly studied, but likely to include the extreme and rapid changes in lifestyle, physical activity and diet that accompany urbanization and rapid economic development. The results of such lifestyle are already being seen. Most cardiovascular disease deaths, generally associated only with Western industrialized countries now occur in developing countries.[2]

Common childhood and adolescent medical consequences of obesity include increased growth, then stunting, increased fat free mass, early menarche, hyperlipidemia, increased heart rate and cardiac output, hepatic steatosis with elevated transaminases and abnormal glucose metabolism.[3,4,5]

The various causative factors attributed to the increasing prevalence of obesity in the Indian scenario may perhaps be attributed to the lifestyle changes of the families. Increased purchasing power, better and comfortable living thanks to the improving technology, increased variety and availability of food products in the market and increased hours of inactivity, have all been blamed for the changing trends. Television, video games and computers have replaced the hours of outdoor games and other activities leading to childhood obesity.

It is thought that the tendency of adults becoming obese is determined by genetic, intrauterine, childhood and adolescent condition. Critical periods for the development of obesity and its sequel have been postulated, including period of gestation, the period of adiposity rebound (between 5-6 years) and adolescence. Studies have also demonstrated that an active life style in childhood is more likely to be reflected in more active adolescents and adults. Although 10 percent weight loss in adults can improve the comorbidities of obesity, most comorbidities are irreversible.[6]

DEFINITION OF CHILDHOOD OBESITY

Obesity actually can be viewed as the energy balance of any individual. Energy expended should be equal to that of energy expended. Therefore, basically it can be defined as energy expended to be equivalent to energy consumed. In other words it means that the energy balance should not be tilted. A positive energy balance will probably lead to overweight and finally obesity.

Overweight and obesity are both labels for ranges of weight that are greater than what is generally considered healthy for a given height. The terms also identify ranges of weight that have been shown to increase the likelihood of certain diseases and other health problems.

For adults overweight and obesity ranges are determined by using weight and height to calculate a number called the body mass index (BMI). BMI is used because, for most people it correlates with their amount of body fat.

An adult with a BMI between 23-24.9 is considered overweight, while one who has a BMI of 25-29.9 is considered obese as per the revised guidelines issued by the Ministry of Health, Govt. of India.

WHAT IS BMI

Body mass index (BMI) is a number calculated from a child's weight and height. It does not measure fat directly, but research has shown that BMI correlates to direct measures of body fat. Moreover it is a simple and inexpensive method of screening for weight categories that may lead to health problems. For children and teens, BMI is age and sex specific and is often referred to as BMI for age.[7]

WHAT IS A BMI PERCENTILE

After BMI is calculated for children and teens, the BMI number is plotted on the CDC BMI-for age growth charts, either for boys or girls, to

Table 2.1: BMI for status categories and percentile

Weight status category	*Percentile range*
Underweight	Less than the 5th percentile
Healthy weight	5th percentile to less than the 85th percentile
At risk of overweight	85th to less than the 95th percentile
Overweight	Equal to or greater than the 95th percentile

(Ref: 7).

obtain a percentile ranking. The percentile indicates the relative position of the child's BMI number among children of the same sex and age. The growth charts show the weight status categories used with children and teens (underweight, healthy weight, a risk of overweight and over- weight).

BMI for age weight status categories and the corresponding percentiles are shown in Table 2.1.

BMI is used as a screening tool to identify possible weight problems for children. CDC and the American Academy of Pediatrics (AAP) recommend the use of BMI to screen for overweight beginning at 2 years of age. It is used to screen for overweight, at risk of overweight, or underweight. But it definitely is not a diagnostic tool. High BMI for age and sex in a child may not necessary determine if excess fat is a problem. For this some other parameters like skinfold thickness measurements, evaluation of diet, physical activity, family histories, etc. are also required.

The BMI for age percentile is used to interpret the BMI number because BMI is both age and sex specific for children and tens. These criteria are different from those used to interpret BMI for adults, which do not take into account age or sex. Age and sex are considered because

- The amount of body fat changes with age
- The amount of body fat differs between girls and boys.

The CDC BMI-for-age growth charts for girls and boys take into account these differences and allow translation of a BMI number into a percentile for a child's or teen's sex and age.[7]

BMI is now a universally accepted standard to measure childhood obesity. A consensus proposed the use of a BMI above the 85th percentile as a screening index for overweight and a BMI above the 95th percentile as an index of excess adiposity in adolescents.[8,9] In other words, when the weight exceeds 110 percent of the standard weight or when the skin fold thickness is more than 30 mm. Obesity is considered when the weight exceeds 120 percent of the standard weight. Super obesity has been described when the weight for height above the 95th percentile on the growth charts from NCHS, and weight in excess of 140 percent of the median weight for a given height.[10]

Measuring skin fold thickness (SFT) can help distinguish patients who are over fat from those who are overweight due to increased muscle and bone. SFT provides direct measure of body fat. It can be measured at several sites, including triceps, biceps axilla, midabdominal, subscapular and suprailiac. SFT above 85th percentile for age and sex suggests obesity and above 95th percentile for age suggests super obesity. The trunk skinfold measurement, subscapular, axilla, suprailiac and abdominal may be suitable indicators of abdominal adipose tissue in children.[11,12]

However, at the Workshop on Childhood Obesity in1999, views from participants were presented, where the use of SFT for measuring obesity in children was debated. It was remarked that the validity of SFT measurement in different populations has not been carefully explored. Further no evidence suggests that SFT measurements predict hyperinsulinemia, hypertension or other illness in children better than does BMI. Results from several data suggest that childhood BMI remains stable into adulthood, better than does SFT. This observation may reflect measurement error in SFT changes in fat distribution.

The group noted that circumference (e.g. waist or hip) may reflect morbidity in adults, but the relation between visceral fat and morbidity in children and adolescents has not been clarified.[13]

PATHOGENESIS OF CHILDHOOD OBESITY

Genetic Factors

Hereditary or genetic factor also has been recognized for obesity. It considers expression of a complex interaction between genetic and environmental factors including food intake. Parental obesity has been considered as a strong predictor, especially when both parents are obese. The resting energy expenditure (REE) and metabolic rate are known to be based on heredity.

Genetic factors have also been linked to birth weight in the pathogenesis of obesity. This has now been recognized as the Barker's theory.[14] This theory is supported by studies suggesting that a low birth weight is adversely associated with a greater risk of cardiovascular disease and type II diabetes in adult life. The relationship between birth weight and adult fatness is affected by many confounding factors, such as gestational age, parental factors and socioeconomic classes.[15]

Many studies have observed that familial aggregation of obesity can be traced through three generations as shown by a report indicating that the grandparents' obesity is related to that of the parents' BMI and also to obesity indices in grand children.[16] It has also been shown that familial factors with regard to eating habits also influence the children's eating behavior and consequently obesity. Similarly, a strong relationship was also found between the level of parental physical activity and that of their preschool children.[17]

Early Feeding vs. Obesity Risk

Scientists have shown that perinatal nutrition is related to obesity risk in young adulthood. In a study during the Dutch famine of 1994-45, significantly lower obesity rates were observed in young adults exposed to famine conditions in the last trimester of gestation and the first months of postnatal life, compared to controls that were not exposed perinatally to the famine.[18]

The feeding of children during the early infancy on breast or formula milk has been found to influence overweight or obesity in them. Previously breastfed children are less likely to be overweight or obese at school entry than children who were previously formula fed. Breastfeeding for at least 6 months was found to be associated with a risk reduction for overweight and obesity of >30 percent and >40 percent respectively.[19]

Metabolic Factors

There can be syndromic obesity which basically is due to certain metabolic diseases. Such obesities are commonly found in children, e.g. Prader-Willi syndrome, Beckwith-Wiedemann syndrome, Laurence-Moon-Biedl-Bardet syndrome, etc.

Environmental/Lifestyle Factors

The most commonly observed form of childhood obesity is due to environmental factors, which are linked to high fat, high sugar foods, junk foods, aerated sweetened beverages, long hours of television viewing or computer/video games and above all sedentary lifestyle.

Other Factors

Constitutional obesity is known in children and perhaps the commonest type. This is basically a result of excess caloric intake.

Endocrine disorders is also known to cause obesity in children, e.g. in Cushing's syndrome or Turner's syndrome. Hypothyroidism and growth hormone deficiency can also lead to obesity.

Polycystic ovarian syndrome is one typical example of obesity in adolescent girls and this is considered to be lined with excess calorie intake also.

There are certain conditions related to neuropsychiatric disorders which can result in obesity. These include bulimia nervosa and other conditions like hypothalamic, pituitary and other brain lesions like craniophyaryngoma. The mechanism involved is thought to be of disregulating appetite.

ASSESSMENT OF OBESITY

The general approach to assess obesity involves:

History

A detailed history is of utmost importance to evaluate obesity. This includes:

- Family history
- Lifestyle pattern
- Dietary history
- Anthropometry
- Laboratory investigations

Family History

It is generally observed that parents of overweight or obese children are also inclined to be overweight or obese. Heredity or genetic factors might have some role in contributing towards obesity in children, as mentioned earlier in this chapter.

Lifestyle Pattern

This is a major contributing factor in the etiology of obesity. Therefore a detailed history of the complete daily routine of the child is essential which includes hours of sleeping, waking, time spent in commuting to school and mode of transport, outdoor activities involving aerobic games, etc. and number of hours of television viewing or involvement in video games. Besides this, frequency of dining out, type of meals taken at school, frequency of celebrations/feasts at home involving food and in between munching are also significant indicators to ascertain their lifestyle.

Dietary History

This involves a detailed dietary intake of the child/adolescent for the whole day.

Anthropometry

Assessing BMI of these children and evaluating them on the growth charts is used to determine them on the growth charts is used to determine the extent of obesity.

Clinical/Laboratory Investigations

These involve bone age which is suggestive of hypothyroidism and may be confirmed by T3, T4 and TSH estimation in serum. A detailed clinical examination can be done which include checking of blood pressure, sugar and lipid profile.

MANAGEMENT OF CHILDHOOD OBESITY

Management of childhood obesity involves multifactor intervention which includes dietary, physical activity, behavioral/psychotherapy, drug therapy and ultimately may be surgical approaches. The factors responsible for the etiology of obesity are also the ones which can be influenced in the treatment or even prevention of obesity. Therefore, exploring the impact of the home environment is crucial to design effective programs to help children establish healthy eating patterns and lifestyle.

Socioeconomic Status (SES)

Socioeconomic status is thought to influence management of obesity indirectly. It is known that adults of lower SES and lower educational qualifications have less healthy diets and are less likely to participate in physical activities like sports. Hence, their children if predisposed to adiposity are likely to live in environments that promote obesity. According to Epstein,[20] if socioeconomic levels are related to parent management success, then families with fewer children also may be of higher SES and may benefit more from parent than do larger families in lower socioeconomic levels. Effective programs emphasize parental attention as an important motivational factor for weight loss. Therefore parental availability is the key to successful management.

Food Consumption and Eating Pattern

It has been worked out that increasing energy intake by as 150 calories per day above the RDA for weight maintenance would result in a significant weight gain over one year.[21]

Besides our social interaction in any sphere of work or area, encourages and facilitates a way of life that promotes weight gain gradually leading to obesity. This imposes a great challenge on the part of the individual to resist or adapt to a criteria of eating behavior to enable them to maintain the required energy balance. Food composition varies from place to place and from family to family. This may also influence adiposity. High fat/sugar diets are generally energy dense and palatable. Therefore, it is important to effectively maintain the energy balance. Food choices need to be strictly monitored. Changes in the recipes can be effected at the same time retaining the palatability. In case of children, care needs to be taken that emphasis is laid on home based diets. This can be facilitated by encouraging home environments to suit the needs of the child's requirements in terms of optimal growth without tilting the positive energy balance. Social events can incorporate home based foods with a variety of food choices and preferences. The increasing culture of dining out in the younger age groups is setting a negative trend with regard to eating behavior. School canteens can be supervised to ensure healthy foods and stress should be made on children getting home packed tiffin. These too can be supervised and monitored by the authorities. Parent teacher meets can be made more meaningful by involving parents in activities like competitions, etc. on healthy packed tiffin. Current dietary recommendations according to American Academy of Pediatrics advocate reducing fat intake and increasing consumption of complex carbohydrates and fiber containing foods including vegetables and fruits.[22]

The early exposure that children have to fruits and vegetables and to foods high in energy, sugar and fats, may play an important role in establishing an hierarchy of preferences and selection. It was shown that children consumed more fruits and vegetables at schools where more of these items were served and the extent to which these are made available and accessible to children may shape their liking for and consumption of these foods.[23]

Food Availability

Generally the access to food is controlled by parents and older siblings. The types of food that are stored at home by them influence the younger child's food consumption and preferences. Therefore parents and elders can be instrumental in providing and facilitating the right type of healthy foods. Junk foods or other energy dense foods should be in restricted access and portion size of such foods if available may be suitably divided. However, when storing the month's ration one should take care to avoid storage of such food which are calorie dense and likely to be a source of temptation for youngsters, and easy susceptibility to obesity.

Food Preferences and Child Feeding Practices

Observations from familial eating patterns suggest that it is the parents who are more likely to over indulge and prompt eating in obese children, compared to the lean ones whose parents are more selective in choosing food varieties for them. Most authors are of the view that children should be allowed to choose from foods that they are offered and control the amounts they choose to eat.[24,25,26]

It has been seen that children are quite responsive to parental attempts to control their intakes. However, it is also established that on the contrary, stringent parental control can exert a negative impact also. They (children) tend to make just the opposite choices and prefer high fat, high calorie foods. Children have also been known to learn to dislike foods when they are encouraged to eat for rewards or when they are bribed into eating. It has been suggested that parental and child feeding practices play a crucial role in the development of individual food preferences and control of food intake.

Social Learning Environment/Early Learning

It is well accepted that the family plays a pivotal role in providing a social learning environment. Certain behaviors, meal patterns and leisure activities that are associated with the development and persistence of obesity are often modeled and reinforced by parents and older siblings at home. Parents who over eat or eat very fast or ignore their internal satiety cue, set a poor example to the children. The onus lies on the parents to present healthy eating styles at home, as well as in external social environments where the family interacts and to model a healthy selection and consumption of foods and regular physical activity. It is a common observation that obese families appear to store more food in all the targeted areas of the home. Since children tend to influence parental habits and even modify them, they can play an active role in the transmission of messages in the home which focus on healthy eating patterns.

The first choice of flavor in a child's diet is either breast milk or formula milk. The perception of flavor in milk also is one of human infant's earliest sensory experiences; and there is evidence to show that this early experience with flavors has an effect on milk intake and later on food acceptance.[27] It has been reported that flavors in breast milk influence infant's consumption. Early experience with a variety of flavors leads to more ready acceptance of new foods later. Studies in rats have shown that because of repeated early experiences with flavors of the maternal diet present in the mother's milk, rat pups learn to prefer their mother's diet. In humans, formula fed infants have experience with only a single flavor, whereas breast fed babies are exposed to a variety of flavors from maternal diet that are transmitted to the milk. It is postulated that varied flavor experience of breast fed infants can facilitate accepted of solid foods during the weaning period, with breast fed infants showing greater initial acceptance of new foods than formula fed infants.[27] Infants and children do not accept new flavors instantly with the exception of sweet or salty foods; but after repeated exposures to new foods, preferences for new foods generally increases, providing increased intakes, although 5-10 exposures may be required.[28]

Physical Activity

Sedentary lifestyle with low activity levels is known to promote childhood obesity. Therefore, increasing physical activity preferably the aerobic type can prove very beneficial in the treatment of obesity in children. Exercise showed a beneficial effect when combined with reduced energy intake programs, dietary and behavioral management techniques or as part of a multicomponent program.[29] Targeting either sedentary behavior or promoting increased physical activity was associated with significant decrease in percent overweight and body fat and improves aerobic fitness. The American Academy of Pediatrics has recommended limiting television viewing to 1-2 hours a day. Limiting television watching and playing video and computer games appears to compel the choice of other pastimes. The couch potato culture among young children and adolescents, if curtailed can give more options and time for them to go for outdoor activities.

Parental Role

The role of parents in making the food choices is also significant. When parents participate actively in their child's weight program, they are expected to modify their own behaviors that contribute to the child's condition and to model eating and exercise behaviors in ways that promote weight loss. They are also expected to work towards accepting new habits and lifestyles. When parents are targeted and provided with reinforcing intervention to promote weight loss, the results are more effective. When parents involved in such programs are supportive and the child motivated enough, long-term success is more likely. Therefore for effective weight loss programs, it is the whole family that should be targeted, rather than just the child alone.

Some authors have found greater success with involving just the parents and excluding the obese child. According to them, this strategy also inculcates healthy eating behavior in the child rather than the conventional dietary interventions that target the child alone.[30,31]

In this model, change is delivered through the parents instead of the obese child. This approach is basically to target a healthy lifestyle and not just weight reduction. This approach seems more rational, since parents are the ones who can play authoritative role models, at the same time provide a family environment, which provides healthy practices related to weight control issues. Moreover it was observed that this approach was more suitable for the young children as compared to the older ones, since the former seem to be more receptive.

Parental involvement without the obese child is thought to help by prompting change in two areas. Firstly, parental cognition and behavior is involved by increasing nutrition/health skills, regular exercise and improved parenting skills. They are encouraged to provide company at meal times and promote participation of all family members in meals. Secondly they are involved to follow regular meal times and scheduled snacks, thereby setting standards for day-to-day eating practice.

Parents are advised to serve meals to the members individually rather than self-helping, teach portion sizes and provide alternate leisure time activities. The second area involves environmental changes so designed to facilitate a healthy lifestyle, rather than relying in individual self-control in eating. They are encouraged to create opportunities for physical activities. Healthy eating is encouraged and inappropriate foods are kept out of reach or sight. At the same time restriction on the amount of food eaten by the child is avoided. The instructions given to parents are:

1. To avoid mixed messages and unintentionally reinforce undesired behavior.
2. To use praise and corrective actions that are directed to the child's behavior rather than pinpointing at his personal attributes.
3. To identify ways to help children develop independence and initiative.
4. To regulate and empower children to make decisions about selected issues and to cultivate friends and outlets in the community.
5. To promote positive attitudes and self-acceptance and to strengthen self-confidence and self-esteem.

CONCLUSION

- Obesity has been recognized as a major public health problem by WHO, but childhood obesity also has posed a equally challenging role for nutritionists and pediatricians. Obese children are at an increased risk of becoming obese adults and the risk is higher if both parents are obese.

- Exclusive breastfeeding in the early months may have a protective role against childhood obesity. Early introduction to a variety of flavors introduced through breast milk can indicate healthy food preferences in the child.
- Education regarding choice of healthy foods, i.e. low fat, low sugars and high fiber foods like fruits and vegetables needs to be imparted from early years of childhood. This can help instill healthy food preferences.
- Management of obesity in children should be with the involvement of the family without focusing on the child in isolation.
- Behavioral and lifestyle modifications with the help of the dietician, pediatrician and a counselor in collaboration with the family can give encouraging results.

REFERENCES

1. Popkin BM. The nutritional transition in low income countries: An emerging crisis. Nutr Rev 1994;52:285-98.
2. Pearson TA. Cardiovascular disease as a growing health problem in developing countries. The role of nutrition in the epidemiological transition. Public Health Rev 1996;24:131-46.
3. Gidding SS, Bao W, Srinivasan SR, et al. Effects of secular rends in obesity on coronary risk factors in children. The Bogalusa Heart study. J Pediatrics 1995;127:868.
4. Arab M. Diabetes mellitus in Egypt World Health Stat Q 1992;45:334.
5. Burns TL, Moll PP, Lanner RM. Increased familial mortality in obese school children: The Muscatine Ponderosity, Family Study, Pediatrics 1992;39:262.
6. Schonfeld-Warden N, Warden CH. Pediatric Obesity. An overview of etiology and treatment. Ped Clinics of N America Apr;1997;vol44(20:339-61
7. National Center for Chronic Disease Prevention and Health Promotion, Division of Nutrition, Physical Activity and Obesity, 2000.
8. Himes JH, Dietz WH. Guidelines for overweight in adolescent prevalence services: Recommendations from an expert committee. Am J Clin Nutr 1994;59:307-16.
9. Must A, Dallal GE, Dietz WH. Reference data for adiposity: 85th and 95th percentiles of body mass index wt/ht^2 and triceps skinfold thickness. Am J Clin Nutr 1999;53:839-46.
10. Kanders BS. Weighing the options. Criteria for evaluating weight management programs. In TPR (Ed):Pediatric Obesity, Washington DC, Academy Press,1995, pg. 210.

11. Brambilla P. Mauzoni P, Simon S, et al. Peripheral abdominal adiposity in childhood obesity. Int J Obe Adol Metab Disord 1994;18:793.
12. Goen MI, Kaskaun M, Shiman WP. Intra-abdominal adipose tissue in young children. Int J Obes Relat Metab Disord 1995;19:279.
13. Mary C, Bellizi, Williams H Dietz. Workshop on Childhood Obesity: Summary of the discussion. Am J Clin Nutr 1999; 70:1735-55.
14. Barker DJ. Fetal origin of cardiovascular disease. Ann Med 1999;31(Suppl.1):3-6.
15. Parsons TJ, Powen C, Logan S, Summerbell CD. Childhood predictors of adult obesity: A systematic review. Int J Obes 1999;23(suppl8):S1-107.
16. Guillaume M, Lapidus L, Beckers F, et al. Familial trends of obesity through three generations, the Belgian-Luxembourg child study. Int J Obes 1995;19:55-9.
17. Moore LL, Lombardi DA White MJ, et al. Influence of parents' physical activity levels or activity levels of young children. J Pediatr 1991;118:215-9.
18. Ravelli ACJ, van der Meulex JHP, Osmond C, et al. Obesity in young men after famine exposure in utero and early infancy. N Engl J Med 1976; 295:349-53.
19. von Kries R, Koletzko B, Saurerwald T, et al. Breastfeeding and obesity: cross sectional study. BMJ 1999;319:147-50.
20. Epstein LH, Koeske R, Wing RR, et al. The effect of family variables on child weight change. Health Psychol 1986;5:1-11.
21. Rosenbaun M, Leibel RL. The physiology of body weight regulation: Relevance to the etiology of obesity in children. Pediatrics 1998;101:525-39.
22. American Academy of Pediatrics. Committee on Nutrition Statement on cholesterol. Pediatrics 1992; 90:469-473.
23. Hearn MD, Baranowski T, Baranowski J, et al. Environmental influences on dietary behavior among children: Availability and accessibility of fruits and vegetables enable consumption. J Health Educ, 1998.
24. Evers C. Empower children to develop healthful eating habits. J Am Diet Assoc 1997;97(suppl 2) :S 116-18.
25. Birch LL. Development of food acceptance in first years of life. Proc Nutr Soc 1998;57:617-24.
26. Birch LL, Fischer Lo. Development of eating behaviors among children and adolescents. Pediatrics 1998;101:539-49.
27. Sulivan SA, Birch LL. Infant dietary experience and acceptance of solid foods. Pediatrics. 1994;93:271-7.
28. Carpretta PI, Petersik IT, Steward AI. Acceptance of novel flavors is increased after early experience of diverse tastes. Nature.1975;254:689-91.
29. Epstein LH, Valoski AM, Vara LS, et al. Effects of decreasing sedentary behavior and increasing activity on weight change in obese children. Health Psychol 1995;14:109-15.

30. Golan M, Weizman A, Apter A, et al. Parents as the exclusive agents of change in the treatment of childhood obesity. Am J Clin Nutr 1998;67:1130-8.
31. Golan M, Fainaru M, Weizman A. Role of behavior modification in the treatment of childhood obesity, with parents as the exclusive agents of change. Int J Obes 1998;22:1217-24.

Chapter 3 Dietary Management in Malabsorption

MALABSORPTION SYNDROME (MAS)

Malabsorption syndrome as the name suggests comprises a syndrome of disorders involving the digestion and absorption in the gastrointestinal tract (GIT). There may be various reasons for this malabsorption. It could be either due to a defect in the functioning or it could be merely functional. This syndrome is characterized by steatorrhea and multiple abnormalities in absorption of nutrients.

Some of the malabsorption disorders which can be modified in response to diet therapy can be grouped into:

1. Abnormalities in the intestinal lumen—*Luminal Phase.*
2. Abnormalities in the mucosa—*Mucosal phase.*
3. Abnormalities in nutrients entering the vascular or lymphatic circulation—*Removal phase.*

Figure 3.1 gives a picture of the various malabsorptive disorders which are responsive to dietary management.

Abnormalities in the Intestinal Lumen

These may be due to:

1. Inadequate lipase hydrolysis, resulting in
   - Pancreatic insufficiency
   - Gastric resection
2. Alteration of bile salt metabolism which may be consequent to
   - Hepatobiliary disease
   - Intestinal resection
   - Bacterial overgrowth

Abnormalities in the Mucosa

These may include :

1. Lactase insufficiency
2. Sucrase isomaltase deficiency

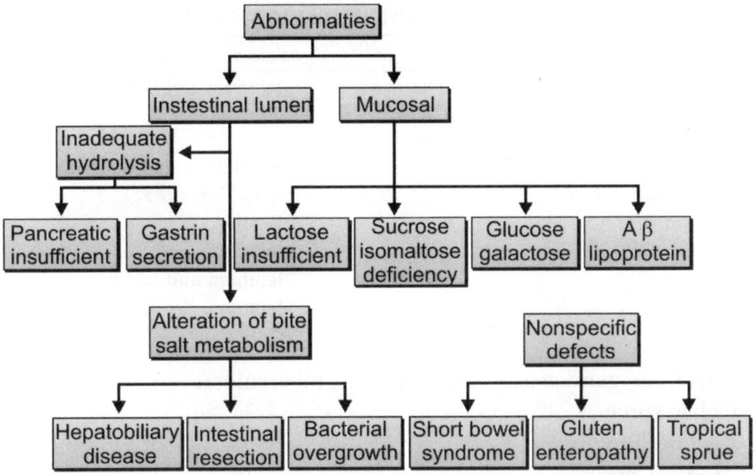

Fig. 3.1: Malabsorptive disorders responsive to dietary modification

3. Glucose galactose deficiency
4. Abetalipoproteinemia

Nonspecific Defects

These may include:
1. Short bowel syndrome
2. Gluten enteropathy
3. Tropical sprue

A child suffering from MAS may present clinically in anyone or more of the following features:
1. Pale, bulky, frothy, foul smelling stools.
2. Stools may be greasy with high fat content and difficult to flush through.
3. There is pronounced wasting and weight loss.
4. Child may present with a distended abdomen.
5. There may be marked features of multiple vitamin deficiencies especially that of B_{12}, iron and folic acid.

There are different sites where different nutrients are absorbed along the whole length of the GI tract. Table 3.1 gives an idea of the absorption of different nutrients at various sites.[1]

Some of the most frequent causes of malabsorption in children in India are:

Table 3.1: Sites of absorption of various nutrients

Nutrients	*Site of maximal absorption*
Proteins, Carbohydrates Lipids, Iron Calcium Zinc, Magnesium, Vitamins A, B_{12}, C, E, K , Folic acid	Jejunum and ileum
Iron, Zinc	Duodenum and Jejunum
Magnesium, Vit. A	Small Intestine
Vitamin B_{12}	Ileum
Folic acid, Vit. D	Jejunum
Vit. E, K, C	Jejunum and Ileum
Water	Jejunum, Ileum and Colon

- Infections-giardiasis, strongyloidiasis, tuberculosis
- Celiac sprue
- Lactose intolerance
- Tropical sprue
- Chronic pancreatitis
- Lymphoma, immunoproliferative small intestinal disease (IPSID)
- Clinically signs which can give evidence of malabsorption may include:
- Progressive weight loss
- Failure to thrive
- Chronic diarrhea
- Steatorrhea (fatty, foul smelling, bulky stool)
- Edema feet
- Weakness, malaise, fatigue
- Abdominal distention
- Excessive flatus
- Abdominal pain
- Symptoms suggesting specific deficiencies, like bleeding, tenderness, muscle cramps, tetany, bone pains
- Symptoms related to cause of malabsorption.

LACTASE INSUFFICIENCY

Lactase is the main carbohydrate present in milk products and comprises a disaccharide consisting of glucose and galactose. Lactose intolerance due to insufficiency of lactase enzyme is the most common form of carbohydrate malabsorption. It is manifested as bloating, flatulence, and or watery diarrhea after ingestion of lactose containing foods. The symptoms are caused by undigested lactose passing from the small intestine into the colon. In the colon the bacteria normally present, ferment unabsorbed lactose, producing short chain fatty acid and gases (carbon dioxide, hydrogen and methane). It is this gas production which causes flatulence, bloating, etc. Unabsorbed lactose also has an osmotic effect in the GI tract draining fluid into the lumen and causing diarrhea. Lactose intolerance can either be primary or secondary.

Primary lactose intolerance could be:

a. Developmental
b. Congenital
c. Late onset

Developmental Lactose Intolerance

This condition can be seen mostly in infants due to the low lactase enzyme present in them. This is because lactase activity develops in the 3rd trimester of pregnancy and in premature birth this enzyme is not fully developed.

Congenital Lactose Intolerance

This is a very rare disorder but if occurs, involves complete omission of milk from the diet.

Late Onset Lactose Intolerance/Secondary Lactose Intolerance

This is also known as adult onset lactose intolerance and is relatively common among Eskimos, native Americans, Asians and some Africans.

Mostly secondary lactose intolerance can be a result of acute diarrhea and is a temporary disturbance of the lactase enzyme. With gradual recovery, the enzyme is also reactivated and the child becomes lactose tolerant again. In infants and toddlers, rotavirus infection commonly leads to lactase deficiency, prompting to withdrawal of milk from the diet of the patient. This condition may also be associated with chronic diarrhea of infancy, food protein intolerance, parasitic infections and gluten-sensitive enteropathy.

The symptoms of secondary intolerance normally disappear once the intestinal wall has recovered from the injury (when the lactase enzyme is restored and reactivated) within 2-4 weeks. Withdrawal of lactose from the diet of the child helps in disappearance of symptoms and reactivates the lactase enzyme.[2]

Actually, the symptoms of lactose intolerance are directly proportionate to the amount of lactose ingested, i.e. the higher the dose of lactose present in the diet, the more severe the symptoms are likely to be. A liter of milk has about 50 g of lactose. Moreover, the dose related tolerance also varies from one child to child and therefore the symptoms may appear in one child even with a lower load of lactose unlike in another who may be tolerant to a slightly higher dose also. This is due to the fact that the metabolic activity of colonic flora varies greatly between different individuals and is believed to play an important role in the presence or absence of symptoms, which are independent of lactase activity in the intestine. Some children and adolescents can tolerate low lactose diets in the form of yoghurt or cereal milk preparations rather than all milk diet. The lactose content of curd is almost 40 percent of that formed in milk.[3] When reintroducing new foods to the diet, recommendation is to wait for 48 hours before each new food or change in amount of food already tolerated.[4]

The feed concentration and quantity can be increased gradually as the child improves clinically. Nutritional supplements and solids are introduced appropriately for the child's age and clinical condition, until the child begins to gain weight. Subsequently, the concentration may be increased by 50-100 percent higher than the normal requirement for actual weight in malnourished children during the period of catch up growth. Care must be taken to keep the osmolality low to prevent osmotic diarrhea.

At times both milk protein and lactose may have to be excluded in cases where there may be milk protein intolerance as a primary cause. In such cases hydrolysed casein products (if commercially available) or sugar milks can be substituted in the diets.

Children who are very sensitive to lactose, need to be careful in choosing foods from the market in readymade form which might contain lactose as a component, e.g. why protein or dried skim milk powder.

A list of some low lactose or lactose free recipes are given below:

LACTOSE FREE RECIPES

Soyabean Milk

Soyabean .... 70 g
Water...................................... 500 ml
Sugar .... 10 g
Salt... a pinch

- Clean soyabean. Soak in water overnight
- Remove skin by rubbing with hands
- Grind it to a fine paste
- Add water and mix thoroughly.
- Filter through a muslin cloth

- Bring to boil. Add sugar and salt
- This gives about 500 ml of milk

Calories: 45/100 ml   Proteins: 2.7 g/100 ml

Soyabean Curd

Soyabean milk .... 250 ml
Curd .... 25 g

- Boil soyabean milk and cool till lukewarm
- Add curd. Mix thoroughly
- Keep it overnight to set.

Calories: 12/100 ml   Proteins: 7.3 g/100 ml

Soyabean Raita

Soya curd .... 250 g
Ripe banana.............................. 2
Sugar .... 50 g
Water.. 25 g

- Mix sugar and water. Bring to boil and cool
- Peel bananas and cut into pieces
- Keep in syrup
- Beat curd well
- Add banana pieces and syrup to beaten curd and serve.

Calories: 540/250 ml   Proteins: 13.9/250 ml

Groundnut Milk

Groundnut kernels................... 100 g
Water.. 600 ml
Sugar .... 12 g

- Soak groundnuts in water overnight
- Remove the red skin by rubbing with hands
- Grind into a fine paste
- Add water and mix well
- Filter through muslin cloth. Use residue in other dishes
- Bring to boil and add sugar
- This gives around 600 ml of milk

Calories: 85/100 ml   Proteins: 3 g/100 ml

Rice and chicken based recipes too may be used for lactose free diets (See also Chapter 4, Tables 4.4 to 4.7)

SUCRASE ISOMALTASE DEFICIENCY

This is a congenital disorder inherited in an autosomal recessive order, with a very rare incidence of 0.2 percent of North Americans and 10 percent of Greenland Eskimos. Symptoms range from severe diarrhea in infancy to intermittent episodes of diarrhea in older children.[4]

Management involves withdrawal of sucrose from the diet of the child, resulting in gradual disappearance of symptoms. Mostly this disorder is limited to the stage of infancy since with age the child generally overgrows the problem.

Trehalase Deficiency

This is an extremely rare disorder. Trehalase is a nonreducing disaccharide commonly associated with plants like mushrooms.

CONGENITAL GLUCOSE GALACTOSE MALABSORPTION

This condition involves malabsorption of glucose and galactose due to a defect in a brush border translocation defect.[5] Symptoms involve the GI tract with profuse diarrhea following ingestion of carbohydrate (dextrose or milk) in the neonatal period. Complete restriction of milk and glucose results in resolving of symptoms. A totally milk free diet needs to be designed with use of fructose instead of glucose.

Sucrose is used in a variety of foods in the form of syrups (medicines), sweets, chocolates, candies, biscuits, etc. Fruits and vegetables contain natural sucrose. Home prepared sucrose free weaning foods can be prepared but commercial baby foods containing biscuits, fruit juices, etc. need to be avoided.

Initially for an infant with sucrose galactose malabsorption, milk substitute should be used in a dilute form, e.g. soyamilk. Feeding may be done in small frequent amounts. The oral rehydration solution used also should be devoid of sucrose. Fructose can be used instead. It may be remembered that fructose being a monosaccharide, feeds containing it can be high in osmolarity compared to glucose polymers (available commercially). Fat emulsions along with fructose can be used to increase the energy density. However, the quantity of fat should not exceed the carbohydrates in the feed. Vitamin and mineral supplements need to be provided separately.

All medicines should be carbohydrate and sorbitol free. Reintroduction of glucose if indicated should be done gradually in patients with temporary or transient intolerance. About 500 mg of calcium per feed or 0.5

percent glucose should be given initially.[6] In case of any adverse reaction, it should be withdrawn immediately. In case it is not tolerated, glucose can be increased gradually over 5-10 days. In case of congenital glucose galactose insufficiency, the child may not tolerate glucose introduction even after several occasions.

ABETALIPOPROTEINEMIA

This is a very rare disorder which affects the absorption of dietary fats, cholesterol and fat soluble vitamins. This is because of the absence of beta lipoproteins which are particles that carry fats and cholesterol in the blood. Due to the absence of these fat carriers, there is reduced absorption of dietary fats and fat soluble vitamins like A, D, E and K from the gastrointestinal tract into the bloodstream.

The signs and symptoms of abetalipoproteinemia appear in the first three months of life. These include failure to thrive, malabsorptive stools involving steatorrhea and impaired functions of the nervous system leading to poor muscle coordination. There may also be involvement of the retina leading to loss of vision. Deficiency of vitamin E is the main cause of these manifestations. Other features might include anemia, abnormal red blood cells, clotting problems, night blindness, poor eyesight and cataract.[7]

Dietary Management

Children diagnosed with abetalipoproteinemia need to have certain dietary modifications, especially with regard to the dietary fat content. Long chain fatty acids have to be restricted and replaced with medium chain triglycerideds like coconut oil. Secondly, the diet needs to be supplemented with the fat soluble vitamins, A, D, E, and K. Appropriate diet planning needs to be done with the help of the dietician to meet the required nutrients for specific age.

REFERENCES

1. Robinson CH. Malabsorption Syndrome. In: Normal and Therapeutic Nutrition. 14th ed Oxford and IBH Publishing Co. pp 466-81.
2. British Nutrition Foundation 2000.
3. Stoker TW, Castle JL. Special Diets In: Walker WA, Watkins JB (Eds). Nutrition in Pediatrics. Basic Science and Clinical Applications, Hamilton, Ontario BC Decker; 1997;771.
4. Ament ME, Perera DR. Sucrose Isomaltase Deficiency-a frequently misdiagnosed disease. J Pediatr 1973;83:721.

5. Wright EM. Genetic Disorders of Membrane Transport. Glucose and Galactose Malabsorption. Am J Physiol Gastrointest Liver Physiol 1998;275:5;879-82.
6. Wimberley PD, Harris JT. Congenital glucose-galactose malabsorption. Proc R Soc Med 1974;67(8):755-56.
7. Berriot-Varoqueaux N, Aggerbeck LP, Samson-Boumatt, Wetterman JR. The role of microsomal triglyceride transfer protein in abetalipoproteinemia. Annu Rev Nutr 2000;20:663-97.

Chapter 4 Nutrition in Diarrheal Diseases

Diarrhea in children can be consequent to infections too besides chronic problems as malabsorption as discussed in Chapter 3. In industrialized societies, this still remains a significant cause of postneonatal morbidity and mortality. It accounts for nearly 40 percent of childhood morbidity and mortality and is highest during the weaning period up to the second year of life. Overcrowding, poor sanitation, and poor feeding hygiene like bottle feeding are the main predisposing factors for acute diarrhea leading to malnutrition.

Based on duration of the diarrhea, we can discuss this problem under 2 categories:

A. Acute diarrhea.
B. Persistent diarrhea.

ACUTE DIARRHEAS (AD)

Acute diarrheas can be a result of acute infections as mentioned earlier in this chapter and is likely to resolve within a few days. But repeated episodes of AD can result in poor appetite, reduced intake and hence reduced absorption of nutrients. Nutritional management therefore is of prime importance to prevent the child from slipping into the cycle of infection and malnutrition.

Nutritional Management of AD

A common practice observed in the developing countries during acute episodes of diarrhea is to withhold feeding. This leads to increased losses which are not able to be met. It also delays the repair of the intestinal mucosa and reversal of digestive enzymes, besides malabsorption of important micronutrients. The concept that feeding increases the stool volume and length of illness is totally unfounded. A number of studies have demonstrated the beneficial effects of early feeding during the course of the illness and the resulting shorter duration of hospital stay.[1,2]

Oral Rehydration Therapy (ORT)

The first step to consider in the management of AD is to tackle the dehydration if existing. ORT is the mainstay of the initial treatment. The oral rehydration solution (ORS) recommended by WHO contains 20 g glucose, sodium chloride, 3.5 g, sodium bicarbonate 2.5 g or sodium citrate 2.9 g and potassium chloride 1.5 g to be mixed in 1 liter of water.[3] However it was found that this composition of ORS proved to be hyperosmolar most of the time since the electrolyte content of noncholera stool is such that, it contains only about 56 mmol/lt of sodium and potassium of about 25 mmol. By using this ORS, a state of hyperosmolarity may be achieved which can only worsen the diarrhea. Some authors have also termed this solution as oral dehydration solution (ODS) instead of ORS.[4] Therefore, it would be prudent to assess the type of diarrhea before choosing the type of ORS. A more user friendly ORS has been formulated-the hypo-osmolar ORS and the super ORS, which is rice based

Among the hypoosmolar solutions available, two are more common:

a. With sodium 75 and glucose 75 mmol/lt.
b. With sodium 60 and glucose 24 mmol/lt

The super ORS solution contains starch 40 g instead of 20 g of glucose per packet.[4] The advantage of using super ORS is that it decreases the stool output by 25 percent, besides avoiding nutrient compromise in the child during the diarrheal episode. Normal feeding is otherwise affected during acute episodes, resulting in significant nutrient losses. By using super ORS which is rice based, some amount of feeding can be ensured. This has been aptly demonstrated by various studies, where a decrease in stool output too was reported by 28 percent and ORS consumption too decreased by 27 percent.[5]

Dietary Management

Adequate feeding during the episodes of diarrhea can not be over emphasized. Anorexia is a common feature observed during any illness but may vary on the type of illness. Febrile illnesses are more prone to lead to decreased intake especially in children. In diarrheal episodes, though there may not be frank anorexia, children and even mothers themselves, prefer to feed only plain liquids more than solids, e.g. water, clear soup, milk, lime juice or even fruit juice. Infants on breastfeeds must be allowed to continue on the same. In fact, it has been demonstrated that infants fed on breast milk during AD, gain weight better and are prevented from going into a state of malnutrition. Moreover, cessation of breastfeeds is known to exert a deleterious effect on the nutritional status of the child, besides increasing the risk of dehydration 5 times as compared to breastfed infants.[6]

In the acute diarrheal episode most children may be lactose tolerant, therefore, withdrawing of milk from their diet should be avoided, unless and until the child has had a history of lactose intolerance earlier. Bhan and his team have had a vast experience on the management of such children and have recommended a calorie intake of at least 125 percent of the normal required with nutrient dense foods and should be continued till the child achieves the preillness weight and normal nutritional status.[7]

WHO has formulated some guidelines for the feeding schedule of infants and children during AD episodes, which is tabulated as in Table 4.1.[8,9]

As evident from this table, stress has been made on continuation of breastfeeds in young infants. This also helps maintenance of lactation in the mother for a longer duration and also ensures better milk production due to the sucking stimulus. For older children or the nonbreastfed infants, animal milk can be offered but, it should be full strength, as soon as dehydration is corrected, as has been advocated by numerous authors.[9,10]

Older children can be fed on a mixed diet of cereal, pulse and vegetables, with addition of oil/ghee/butter for increasing the density without increasing the bulk. Milk cereal combinations are also well tolerated

Table 4.1: Feeding during acute diarrhea

Stage of hydration and feeding pattern	*Recommended schedule of feeding*
A. During rehydration phase	
• Breastfed Infants	Continue breastfeeds
• Nonbreastfed infants	preferably give ORS till rehydration. Beyond 4 hours, animal milk/food
• In severely malnourished children	offer some food as soon as possible
B. After rehydration phase	
Breast fed infants	continue breastfeeds more frequently
Non breast fed infants	offer undiluted animal milk/formula as before
Infants 4-6 months	add energy dense cereal/pulse supplements
Older children	give energy dense thickened feeds with oil-pulse (K rich) and green leafy vegetables, carrots, etc. encourage feeding 6 times a day

(WHO, 1991).

even among the slightly lactose intolerant children. Amylase rich factor (ARF) can be made use of to reduce the viscosity of the feeds.

NUTRITIONAL MANAGEMENT OF PERSISTENT DIARRHEA

Persistent diarrhea (PD) or protracted diarrhea is defined when the duration of passage of stools exceeds 14 days. The state of hydration may or may not be preserved. Growth faltering and severe malnutrition are characteristic features in this condition. This is due mainly to inadequate intake and in most cases with malabsorption.

PATHOGENESIS OF PERSISTENT DIARRHEA

The pathogenesis in PD may involve digestion and absorption of all the nutrients—carbohydrates, proteins and fats.

In carbohydrate malabsorption usually there is disaccharide deficiency due to the decreased luminal amylase resulting in impaired exocrine pancreatic function. Lactose enzyme is the one which is mostly affected, leading to secondary lactose intolerance. This condition is frequently encountered following rota viral diarrheas where the villous tip cells are partially damaged. Lactose enzyme being the first to be affected is also the last to be restored for adequate absorption of lactose.

Sucrase enzyme too can be affected leading to malabsorption of sucrose in protracted diarrheas. These can lead to ineffective villous repair or prolonged mucosal injury in malnourished children. This in fact also can be the cause of PD.

Steatorrhea is often associated in PD due to insufficient pancreatic lipase or due to the defect in bile acid metabolism. Similarly protease activity in the pancreatic secretion may also be compromised, especially in children with PD.

Cow's milk protein intolerance (CMPI) is sometimes associated with PD and can be seen in children below 6 months of life. The β-lactoglobulin fraction in cow's milk is the cause for CMPI in such children. Milk antibody and IgE are increased in the mucosa in this condition, and this itself can lead to PD also. Such children may also be known to be intolerant to soya protein and may present with blood and mucus.

Finally, PD can also result from abnormal bacterial colonization in any part of the gastrointestinal tract. Breastfed babies are however prone to be protected from such attacks. It is mostly the older children who are on mixed diet or formula feds, who may be affected by such over growth of bacteria. Common examples are the *Clostridium difficile* and bacteriodes.

DIETARY MANAGEMENT

As emphasized earlier, infants below 6 months already on breastfeeds should be continued on the same. Older infants will however not be satisfied with breast milk alone nor will their nutritional needs be met with only breast milk.

Dietary manipulation in older children presenting with diarrhea depends upon the malabsorptive state of the child. They may be partially lactose intolerant to sucrose besides lactose. Children presenting with PD generally might already have been fed on milk based diets for the first week or ten days. In such children the lactose load can be decreased by substituting curd for milk or buttermilk too can be offered also. For older infants beyond 6 months, cereal and milk based formulae can be used where the total quality of milk used is quite less. Rice is the most preferred cereal used. Rice can be made into flour which makes it easier to cook into porridge or gruel form. Some of the formulae used have been recommended by the Indian Academy of Pediatrics as shown in Tables 4.2 and 4.3. These provide approximately 80 cals./100 ml and about 2.5 g/100 ml of protein.

These feeds can be given by nasogastric route also in cases where oral feeding is difficult to achieve. It is generally observed that children who are difficult to feed and are put on tube feeding, generally regain their appetite within 5-6 days and if oral feeding is restored over a period of time nasogastric feeds can be stopped.

Table 4.2: Low lactose diets for infants (milk with rice) (4-12 months)

Ingredients	*Amount*	*Calories (%)*	*Proteins (g %)*
Milk	75 ml	52	2.6
Rice	5 g	17	0.4
Sugar	2.5 g	10	-
Water	100 ml		
Total		79	3

Lactose content-4.5 g percent.
(IAP, 2006).

Table 4.3: Curd with rice feed

Ingredients	*Amount*	*Calories (%)*	*Protein (g %)*
Curd	75 ml	45	2.3
Rice	5 g	17	-
Sugar	2.5 g	10 ml	-
Water	100 ml	72	2.7

At this stage, the feeds can be made slightly thicker, to make them more calorie dense, by either increasing the amount of cereal or addition of oil proportionately. Coconut oil, a good source of medium chain triglyceride (MCT), can be used successfully to avoid further deterioration of malabsorption. Older children can be given a mixed cereal pulse based family diet, e.g. 'khichdi', which is traditionally used even otherwise in Indian families. Banana is a good calorie dense supplement and also potassium rich, and hence can be used for most children.

There are also a considerable percentage of children who may not tolerate lactose based and may need to be taken off milk/curd completely. This is evident from the perianal excoriation seen in children with continuous purging. In such cases, a total milk/curd free feed is advised, where in cereal pulse based diets like blenderized khichdi can be fed. Somc of these feeds are shown in Tables 4.4 and 4.5.

Egg white based feeds along with rice powder, glucosc and oil has also been formulated by WHO,[10] but in the Indian context, due to certain religious and cultural constraints, it may not be well accepted.

Only rice based formulae should be used for infants below 6 months of age at this stage. The gut malnutrition in terms of enzymes is more efficient after the age of 6 months and secondly too early introduction of variable proteins may also lead to hypersensitization in some cases. Rice is considered the least allergenic among the cereals, therefore, it is better to begin first with rice based feed alone and then gradually add other protein sources. An example of rice based formula is given in Table 4.6. This formula is slightly low in calories and also in proteins, but the

Table 4.4: Lactose free diets
cereal pulse based feeds (sweet)

Ingredients	*Amount*	*Calories (%)*	*Protein (g %)*
Rice	15	48	1.2
Moong dal	5	17	1.1
Sugar	2.5	10	-
Oil	2.5	22	-
Water	100	97	2.3

Table 4.5: Cereal pulse based feeds (salty)

Ingredients	*Amount*	*Calories (%)*	*Proteins (g %)*
Rice	4.0 g	13.8	2.7
Moong dal	6.0 g	21.0	14.7
Oil	5.0 ml	45.0	-
Water	100 ml	80	1.7

Table 4.6: Rice gruel (sweet)

Ingredients	*Amount*	*Calories (%)*	*Proteins (%)*
Rice	5.0 g	17	0.3 g
Sugar	4.5 g	18	4
Oil	3.0 g	27	-
Water	100 ml	62	0.3

Table 4.7: Comminuted chicken feed

Ingredients	*Amount (g)*	*Calories*	*Proteins (g)*
Chicken	100	110	26
Glucose	50	200	-
Coconut oil	50	440	-
Water	1000	750	26

(Per 100 ml of feed contains 75 cal. and 2.6 g of protein).

energy can be increased by addition of more oil, preferably MCT, and the protein content can be enhanced by addition of any commercially available protein supplement like protinex. Most of the supplements available are skim milk based, therefore care should be taken to read the labels before using them in such feeds. Other lactose free commercial supplements available are soyal, prosoyal, zerolac nusobee and Simyl MCT. These contain in addition some essential micronutrients, like vitamins and minerals and varying amounts of taurine, carnitine and MCT.

It has been observed that some children, who are lactose intolerant, are also intolerant to soya protein, and therefore these children can not be offered such feeds. In such situations, the only option left is to use rice based feeds and pulses can be added in older infants comminuted chicken feeds may also be tried.

A small percentage of infants may not respond to even lactose free diets as they may be intolerant to sucrose also. In such cases, lactose and sucrose free formulae have to be used which are available commercially. These have been tried successfully in many centers.

Some centers also use comminuted chicken for lactose and sucrose free diets (Table 4.7), but due to religious issues, these are not very commonly popular.

Once the child is put on any of the above-mentioned feeds, the quantity can be gradually increased. Small frequent feeding, about 5-6 times a day helps ensure adequate nutrient intake and also in faster recovery. Older children can be fed with the home based solid diets without including lactose. It may be borne in mind, that once the child slips into a state of PD, the recovery also is a slow process. The lactose enzyme which is the first to be affected is also the last to return to normalcy. It is usually about 4-6 weeks by the time lactose foods can be reintroduced successfully. Therefore, low lactose diets may first be introduced, like curd, which can be tried initially and gradually milk based porridge or gruels can be initiated. The amounts may be small first and gradually increased as tolerance improves.

In case if a child with chronic or intractable diarrhea fails to respond to the above regimen, parenteral nutrition (PN) needs to be considered. The major part of energy is provided by the fat emulsion mixture, containing essential fatty acids. However, PN has its own disadvantages, if used over a prolonged period. Hence, it should be given only till the oral intake is restored.

REFERENCES

1. Brown KH, Gastanaduy AS, Saavedra JM, et al. Effect of continued oral feeding on clinical and nutritional outcomes of acute diarrhea in children. J Pediatr 1998;112:191-200.
2. Ornestein SR. Enteral vs. parenteral therapy for intractable diarrhea of infancy. A prospective randomized trial. J Pediatr 1981;99:360-61.
3. Mahalanbis D, Bhan MK. Development of an improved oral rehydration solution, Ind J Pediatr 1991;58:757-61.
4. KE Elizabeth. Diet in various diseases, In: Nutrition and Child Development. 3rd Ed; pg 224-230. Paras Medical Publishers.
5. Molla AM, Ahmed SM, Greenough WB III. Rice based oral rehydation solution decrease the stool volume in acute diarrhea. Bull WHO 1985;63:7556.
6. Faraque AS, Mahalanabis D, Islam A, Hoque SS, Hasnat A. Breastfeeding and oral rehydration at home during diarrhea to prevent dehydration. Arch Dis Child 1992;67:1027-9.
7. Arora NK, Bhan MK. Nutritional management of acute diarrhea. Ind J Pediatr 1991;58:763-7.
8. Jelliffe DR, Jelliffe EFP. Dietary management of young children with acute diarrhea, 2nd Ed. Geneva, WHO, 1991;3-26.
9. World Health Organisation. The management and prevention of diarrhea. Practical Guidelines. 3rd Ed. Geneva,WHO,1993;1-4.
10. Bhan MK, Arora NK Khoshoo V, et al.Comparison of a lactose free cereal based formula and cow's milk in infants and children with acute gastroenteritis. J Pediatr Gastroenterol Nut 1998;7:208-13.

Chapter 5

Diet in Celiac Disease

Celiac disease (CD) was first described in 1950 by Dicke in Holland[1] by chance observation that during the German occupation when food availability was scarce and poor nutrition, children kept better health. Subsequently, with improved nutrition, when wheat was more liberally available, children actually deteriorated in health. This set him to infer that perhaps it was the wheat which was the culprit, the introduction of which could cause features of malabsorption. The classical histopathological description of the disease was given by Paulley in 1954.[2] Other cereals like barley, wheat and rye were also identified around the same period to cause CD. By 1960, it was also identified in India and perhaps for the first time reported by Walia et al.[3] In 1979, Walker-Smith described it as a disease of the proximal small intestine characterized by an abnormal small intestine mucosa and associated with permanent intolerance to gluten. Removal of gluten from the diet leads to a full clinical and pathological remission.[4]

INCIDENCE

CD was earlier known to occur in the predominantly wheat eating areas like Europe, Australia and North America. It was first thought to be around 1 in 3000 in England but over a period of time, it was observed by Mylotte in the West Ireland that the incidence could be as high as 1 in 300.[5]

However, Asian countries like India too are not spared of this entity, and there are reports from the Middle East in Arab children as well. Reports of CD from the Northern India have shown a remarkable steady increase over a time period. His could be partly attributed to the fact that there is growing awareness regarding the existence of this entity among the clinicians as compared to what was true about a couple of decades ago. Genetic factors are also known to predispose to gluten hypersensitivity as the disease is also known as. The condition may occur in one or member of the same family. Reports of concordance for CD in monozygotic twins are also available.[6]

PATHOGENESIS—*WHAT IS GLUTEN?*

Gluten is the protein fraction of found in wheat. It is a large complex molecule that has been divided chemically into four hetrogenous proteins-gliadins, glutenins, albumins and globulins. In CD, it is the gliadin fraction of gluten which is responsible for the pathogenesis. This gliadin itself is a complex protein consisting of 40 different components. The alpha-gliadin is the main toxic entity of the gluten, though it has also been associated with a small peptide. The beta-gama, and omega-gliadin are also known to be toxic in nature. Other cereals found to be toxic are rye, barley and oats. But the inclusion of barley and oats as gluten free are controversial with different authors reporting diverse opinions. Barley contains the protein hordein, which is also known to cause mucosal changes when given in highly artificial circumstances.[7]

It was suggested during later years that the amount of gliadin present in the nominally gluten free products may be significant in very sensitive patients. In 1979, WHO proposed a standard for the permitted residual protein in a wheat (or other gluten containing cereal), starch based gluten free product of not more than 0.3 percent protein in dry matter and the proposed regulations require that the total nitrogen content of wheat, rye or barley, etc. used in gluten free products should not exceed 0.05 g per 10 g of these grains on a dry matter basis and that the nature of the source of the starch should be declared on the label.[8]

The mechanism leading to damage in the intestine is:

- It is caused by an immune response to gluten containing diet
- Factors facilitate the gluten induced injury
- Incomplete digestion of gluten due to deficiency of enzymes results in the accumulation of toxic substances that damage the mucosa
- Toxicity is mediated by a lecithin like interaction between gluten and intestinal epithelial cells.[9,10]

More recently CD is considered as an autoimmune reaction to the tissue transglutaminase in the intestinal mucosa initiated by exposure to dietary gluten in genetically predisposed individuals. It is a symptomatic or symptom free disease, closely associated with risk allelels on the human leukocyte antigen (HLA) class 11 genes and it may develop at any age during childhood or adulthood.[11]

CLINICAL FEATURES OF CD

Diagnosing CD in a child may not always be a straight forward process since there may be variable signs and symptoms. Most of these like recurrent diarrhea or not gaining weight may be overloaded and not given due significance by parents themselves. The former problem may be treated off and on for infections and in a peripheral set up, and the failure to gain weight is often overlooked by parents and hence delaying seeking of medical attention. At times in the absence of diarrhea or failure to thrive, the child may always appear pale and the parents may fail to observe it. The initial signs of mild-to-moderate anemia are hardly noted by parents and only when he child probably presents with complaints of weakness, fatigue or loss of appetite, do the parents seek medical help. Even if they are in some remote area not accessible to some medical centre, they may be treated with some hematinics or appetite boosters or some multi vitamin supplememts. Therefore to diagnose CD, it is important that the health caregivers think along the lines of features of malabsorption. Only then would an attempt be made to work up for ruling out CD.

The common symptoms suggestive of CD are:

- Steatorrhea: Almost 70 percent of children suffering from CD present with pale bulky, offensive stools. A close look at the stool may also reveal small fat globules sticking around.
- Failure to thrive: Often children with CD may present with failure to gain weight despite reasonable intake, and may show features of wasting. At times some may otherwise appear normal but parents may complain of the child appearing smaller for his age as compared to his peers. Pot belly is a typical feature in these children.
- At times in the absence of any of the above symptoms, parents may just present a child for not eating adequately or loss of appetite, lethargy or easy fatigueability even without much exertion. A routine examination may reveal severe anemia and on further work up for one of the differential diagnosis, the child may prove positive for CD. The anemia in these children is generally of the iron deficiency type rather than the megaloblastic one, though blood folate levels may also be reduced.[12]
- Skin Manifestations: Some of the children with CD may present with skin manifestations like knuckle pigmentation and skin infections. Dermatitis herpetiformis is commonly observed in such children.
- Others: Symptoms like vomiting, pain abdomen, irritability, constipation or rectal prolapse in some may also be found in children with CD.
- The European Society for Pediatric Gastroenterology and Nutrition (ESGAN) in 1970 evolved definite criteria to label a child with CD.[13]

These include:

a. It is a permanent condition.
b. There is a flat mucosa in upper and small intestine.
c. There has to be a biochemical evidence of malabsorption, but some of them may be asymptomatic at the time of investigation.
d. A gluten free diet (GFD) results in complete restoration of mucosal architecture and tests for malabsorption also become normal.
e. Later introduction of gluten into the diet will be followed by recurrence of the mucosal abnormalities. There may or may not be clinical symptoms for months and years.

DIAGNOSTIC CRITERIA

To diagnose CD a variety of tests are used which can decide further course of management in a child with CD. It should be kept in mind that since the mainstay of management in treating CD is dietary therapy alone, which means withdrawal of gluten from the child's diet and since gluten is the primary component of any diet especially in the Northern India, it can come as a great shock to the parents once diagnosis is confirmed to them and the management explained.

The various diagnostic criteria include:

a. Stool Test- a 24 hour fecal fat test is done to establish the extent of fat malabsorption.
b. D-Xylose test
c. Breath hydrogen test
d. Intestinal biopsy challenge tests.

AGE OF PRESENTATION

In an Indian setting the age of presentation of CD in a child is generally after the age of 2 years and more since it is by this age in most communities that the child is more or less totally weaned to a complete solid diet comprising mainly wheat and wheat products. However children between the ages of 10-18 months also are introduced to certain wheat products, mainly in the form of biscuits or suji kheer, but the amount of gluten exposure during this age may be very low and secondly by the time the clinical signs begin to present and parents concerns are aroused, the child may already have reached 2 years or more. As mentioned earlier in the initial stages, recurrent diarrhea or failure to gain weight may be treated as common infections by physicians too. There are reports of CD presenting between ages 1-5 years by some authors.[14]

MANAGEMENT (GFD)

After thorough work up and investigation, if a child is proven to test positive for CD, the next step is the biggest challenge on the part of the clinicians and the dieticians, that of management.

Dietary management is 'the only' management in a child with CD. Gluten withdrawal is the mainstay of management of such children. A typical North Indian diet comprises mainly gluten in all or at least part of the day's diet.

In gluten free diet, i.e. foods totally devoid of wheat and wheat products, rye barley (jaun) and oats, needs to be excluded from the diet completely. Regarding oats, there are controversies of its being safe to include or exclude. But most dieticians to be on the safe side and to avoid any benefit of doubt prefer to advise complete exclusion from the diet. The dictum 'when in doubt discard' holds true in this context. On the face of it, to counsel the parents to stop gluten in the child's diet seems simple enough, but practically when we are faced with such situations, it has been observed that the initial reaction of the parents is that of shock, denial and disbelief. In the predominantly wheat consuming States, like Punjab, Uttar Pradesh, Himachal Pradesh, Haryana and Madhya Pradesh, one cannot even imagine of a day's diet without wheat in some form or the other.

In our day-to-day life we would observe that wheat and its by products like 'suji', 'dalia', 'sewain' are commonly used in preparations like biscuits, snacks, sweets and even daily meals. There are ahost of foods available outside the home which children tend to consume, e.g. breads, biscuits, cakes, pastries or any other bakery products, snacks like 'samosas',' mathi', 'pakoras' and many other savoury products categorized as 'namkeen'. Exclusion of gluten implies a full stop to all these food items. This comes as a rude shock to the parents and a number of times more than the child it is the parents who go into depression and seem visibly upset over the realization of the impact of treatment of their child. A list of foods that are allowed and restricted are given in Table 5.1.

It is here that the dietician's role of counseling comes in and it is indeed a challenge for him or her to convince the parents that there are a host of other alternative foods from which the child has the liberty to choose from, without compromising his growth and development as can be seen from Table 5.1. Soya flour gram flour, rice flour, corn flour and arrowroot flour are some of the other alternative which can be included into the diets of these children. (See Annexure 1 for GFD recopies).

Table 5.1: Foods to be excluded in gluten free diets

- All wheat based products: wheat flour, maida, suji (semolina), oats, barley, rye.
- All bakery products like biscuits, rusks, cakes and pastries buns from maida, suji or wheat flour.
- Baby foods like cerelac, etc.
- Beverages like horlicks, bournvita, protinex and other products where 'malt' word is shown on the labels of the packings.
- All sauces, creams, pie fillings, chocolates, flavored milk shakes, yogurt, where gluten may be present in indirect form.
- Ready to eat flavored crisps, e.g. MacDonalds' chips, etc.
- Meat products like sausages, hamburgers, tinned meat products, fish fingers, etc. where bread crumbs may be used.
- Malt vinegar, soy sauce, spreads, etc.
- Cooking oils (mixed vegetable oil) can contain wheat germ oil, so ensure that oil used is free of it or else sunflower or olive oil can be used safely.
- Beer and whisky are made from grain containing gluten but other alcoholic drinks like wine and cider can be used which is gluten free.
- Some medicines contain gluten which needs to be checked with the chemist or clinician.
- Vegetable gum
- Noodles and pizza, etc.
- Modified food starch, hydrolyzed protein like in 'protinex'.

Table 5.2: Foods that can be included

- Dairy products like milk (fresh, tinned, powder), butter, cream
- Meat, fish and poultry
- All green vegetables, roots and tubers
- All fruits, dried fruits and nuts
- All pulses and legumes like peas, beans, etc.
- Maize, rice, soya flour, gram flour, jowar, bajra, ragi, waterchestnut ('singhara flour')
- Tapioca, sago arrowroot
- Potato flour
- Beverages like tea, coffee, fresh juices, fizzy drinks gelatin, etc.
- Custard powder
- Gluten free flours and cereals available commercially but certified.

The parents have to be reassured that excluding gluten from the diet will not be as difficult as may appease to them. On the contrary that they should be reassured that this treatment implies restriction of only a particular variety of food item and no other medicine or surgical intervention is required. They have to be made to understand that dietary modification is 'the only' treatment for CD and with good compliance the child can lead a healthy normal life just like his peers. Regular follow-up visits are very important for these parents and children and a close rapport between them will help the child understand the significance of dietary restrictions. The parents need to be explained the long-term prognosis of this disease, stressing the importance of such modifications for life without intending to scare them unduly.

Children with CD need not be restricted to go out for social get-togethers where eating is a part of the function, but of course he needs to be explained if he is old enough, what food can be taken safely, e.g. milk, curd preparations, rice and other rice based recepies, fruits or fruit juices and candies, etc. At the same time, it is a good idea if the hostess is aware of such special needs of her guests so that she may be able to include some alternative dish which this child can safely partake. Alternatively they can carry their own tiffins in case they are on a trip outside. Now a days there are some gluten free cereals available in some super markets from where mothers can procure them and plan recopies accordingly. The culinary skills of the mothers with some innovative ideas can help break the monotony of the diet of the child with CD.

GOALS OF NUTRITIONAL THERAPY

1. To achieve the nutritional requirements in terms of macro and micronutrients.
2. To ensure a balanced diet for the desired age.
3. To ensure compliance to GFD.
4. To monitor growth and development periodically-regular follow-up visits.
5. To look for and prevent any associated complications.

The above goals can be achieved as follows:

- The nutritional requirements can be calculated on the basis of age and weight of the child. Most often since these children had been anorexic, their intake would have been very poor. Therefore it would be aimed to begin with a minimum of 100 calories/Kg body weight and gradually build up to 200 calories over a period of time. Proteins can be around 1 g/Kg body weight since lower than this is not always practical as most of the caloric dense foods in a mixed diet would also be rich in proteins, e.g. cereals, pulses and milk and milk products. It can be gradually increased to 1.5-2 and even 3 g/Kg depending upon the appetite of the child as he recovers. Fat content of the diet may vary from 25 percent to as high as 40 percent of the total calories, depending upon the need to meet the calorie requirements. Moreover on a gluten free diet there are certain recipes which may require slightly higher ratio of fats in their preparations. Other nutrients may be supplemented as per the requirement based on clinical or bio chemical parameters from time to time.

- Having decided upon the requirements, efforts should be made to plan the day's menu such that there is variety and at the same time balanced in terms of all the food groups to be provided.
- Compliance on a gluten free diet is the mainstay in such children. The earliest signs of recovery on GFD are evident by apparent cheerfulness of the child, his appetite returns and looks more alert and takes interest in the surroundings. Weight gain comes much later. It has been noticed that most often where compliance is poor, the parents or other elders in the family have been responsible for it. They might be inclined to give 'a little' of any gluten based diet once in a while, thinking that it will not make much of a difference. This can happen especially in an environment where the literary level of the parents might be low or even in the lower socioeconomic strata, where it might be difficult for them to adhere to the restrictions in the absence of availability of alternative foods. Also, it may be due to paucity of time available with the mother to cook separately for this child or due to certain family pressure they may not be able to provide alternative foods to such children. In some cases, despite parental compliance and effort, the child may on the sly share some food with his peers or other siblings. All these factors need to be borne in mind and strict supervision should be maintained for optimum compliance.
- The children are called on a regular follow-up visits and monitored for their growth and any other related clinical signs. Initially their visits may be monthly, gradually relaxing to quarterly, six monthly and then annually depending on their progress. This also ensures compliance and reassurance to the parents and the child to maintain on GFD. A good rapport can be built with them and any doubts regarding the choice of foods can be dealt with them from time to time. If required protein supplements may be advised in case of vegetarian children who may also be lactose or milk intolerant.
- In a few cases there may be presence of certain other factors like diabetes or lactose intolerance or cow's milk protein intolerance which could be a part of complications of gluten enteropathy as the disease is also known. Such conditions may have to be tackled accordingly. Careful selection of various food items allowed or disallowed keeping in mind the lactose containing foods or restrictions imposed for the diabetic state also.

ADHERANCE TO GED

After counseling sessions on GFD to the parents and the children, the next step is to assess the adherance. This can be done by maintaining regular follow-up records in terms of anthropometry, dietary intake or any other visible signs and symptoms. Failure to gain the desired weight and height can be an alert to suspect noncompliance in any form. This can be assessed by obtaining a detailed dietary history from the parents or a 24-hour dietary recall may be taken regarding the various foods taken in the recent past. Indirect probing from the child regarding his or her activities at home or school or time spent with peer groups may give a clue of the kind of foods he could have access to or would be taking inadvertently. There are a number of food categories which might have gluten in some latent or indirect form which otherwise might be considered gluten free, e.g.

- Sweets made from milk, khoya, paneeer which might have some amount of suji or maida mixed by unscrupulous manufacturers. Products containing malt in any form like chocolates. Health supplements, e.g. horlicks, bournvita, protinex, etc.
- Creams, soups and gravies which might have maida or thickening agents
- Any processed food products when specific labeling is not indicated.
- Inadvertent contamination of gluten free cereals like maize, gram flour or rice flour with residue of wheat products during the processing or milling in a mill
- Any medicines, gums or toothpaste might have some gluten as a base ingredient
- Any 'prasad' from religious places even though taken in very minute quantities
- Social eating especially in outdoor catered foods where one may not be sure of the ingredients used in any unstandardized recipes.

Duration of Treatment/Follow-up

As per the definition criteria of ESPGAN, GFD needs to be considered for life, i.e. it is usually for life, even though the patient remains asymptomatic. This is because, it is expected that on a GFD, chances of complications or late recurrences can be avoided, e.g. chronic deficiencies, infertility, etc. which could be associated with gluten sensitivity. Walker-Smith had laid down criteria for the duration on which to keep a child on GFD (Fig. 5.1), and then give a gluten challenge to determine the response. Based on this response, normal or abnormal mucosa on a biopsy after giving a gluten challenge can help to determine whether GFD needs to be continued or can be stopped safely without chances of relapse.

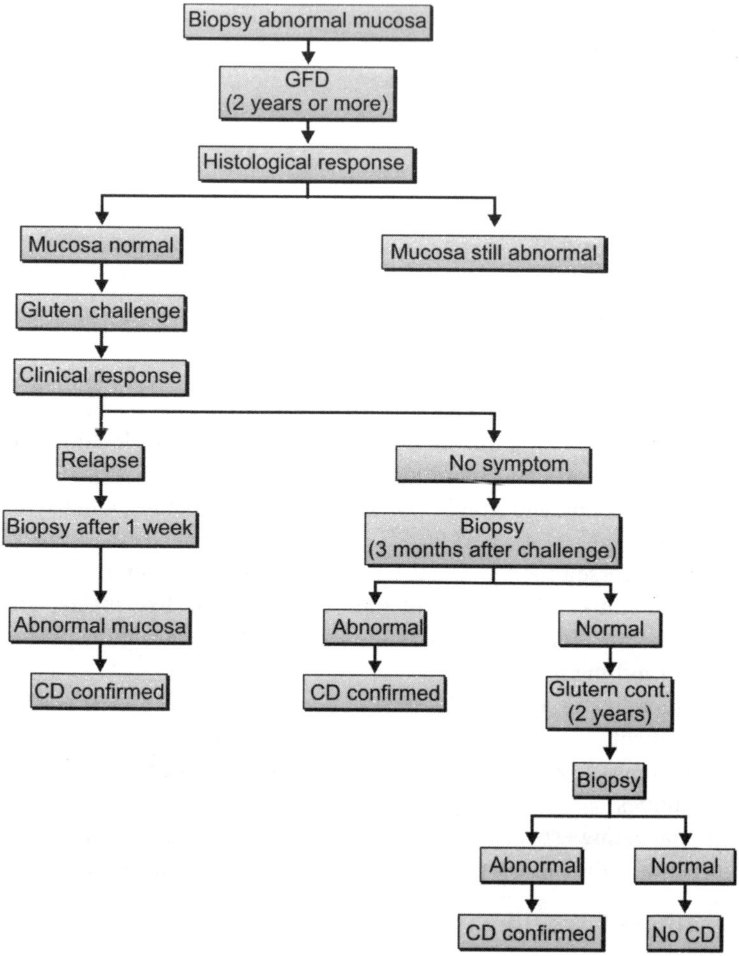

Fig. 5.1: Diagnostic Criteria and investigation for celiac disease (Walker-Smith, 1979)[4]

GLUTEN CHALLENGE

The Working Group of the World Congress of Pediatric Gastroenterology, Hepatology and nutrition in 2002[15] have recommended gluten challenge and subsequent biopsies in children where:

- Initial biopsy was performed before 2 years of age
- Initial diagnosis is doubtful
- Noncompliant patients

- Asymptomatic individuals detected through screening program
- Patient desires a gluten challenge.

However, it is opined that gluten challenge should be avoided during the growth period of a child till up to puberty, to avoid the risk of a set back in the velocity of development in the event of exacerbation of symptoms. Challenge may be given by introduction of 10-20 g of gluten in a phased manner or just allowing the child to have a normal diet as the whole family which would include wheat, may be in the form of chapattis, biscuits or any other wheat based preparation.

FACTORS AFFECTING GLUTEN SENSITIVITY

- **Time of Gluten Introduction:** It is speculated that the timing of exposure of gluten into the child's diet might also have a bearing on the manifestation of symptoms of gluten sensitivity. Norris et al[16] in 2005 have shown links between early infant diet and development of celiac disease. According to their studies in 1560 children it was observed that the initial exposure to gluten in the first 3 months or at 7 months and later significantly increased the risk of CD as compared with exposure at 4-6 months. They had defined CD autoimmunity by the presence of tTG autoantibodies or small bowel biopsy evidence of crypt hypoplasia or villous atrophy. Increased risk was defined as having first degree relative with Type I diabetes or the presence of HLA-DR3, alleles, genes that are associated with an increased risk of autoimmune disease. They therefore concluded that the timing of first gluten exposure is associated with the appearance of CD autoimmunity in children at increased risk for the disease.
- **Amount of Gluten:** It has been postulated that the amount of gluten ingested could be as important as the timing if gluten introduction. This has been demonstrated by Weile et al[17] where a profound difference in the prevalence of CD exists between Denmark (a very low) and Sweden (high prevalence). The explanation given was a remarkable difference in the diet of infants who actually receive much less gluten in Denmark. In Sweden an epidemic of CD was observed which was related to rapid increase in the consumption of gluten at 6 months of age.[18]
- **Breastfeeding and the Time of Gluten Introduction:** In a Swedish study on 627 children with risk of CD exposed to gluten compared to 1254 controls, it was found that the risk of symptomatic CD before 2 years of age was reduced in children if they were breastfed at the time of introduction of dietary gluten.[19]

A systematic review and meta analysis of observational studies published between 1996 and June 2004,[20] revealed that breastfeeding may offer protection against the development of CD. Breastfeeding during introduction of dietary gluten and duration of breastfeeding were associated with reduced risk of developing CD. However, it was not clear whether breastfeeding delays the onset of symptoms or provides permanent protection against the disease.

Breast milk may reduce the risk of CD in childhood through its protective immune components including secretory IgA. On the other hand, the protective effect of breast milk may modulate gluten introduction, resulting in a less rapid or a reduced amount of dietary gluten in the infant diet.

COMPLICATIONS OF CELIAC DISEASE

The National Institute of Health (NIH) in 2004 warned of the following complications of celiac disease if left untreated:

- **Malnutrition:** If not treated or partially treated children with CD show signs of failure to thrive, anemia and multiple vitamin deficiencies resulting in fatigue, stunted growth, neurological problems, low bone density and malabsorption.
- **Osteoporosis/Ostopenia:** In untreated celiac, there are losses of calcium and vitamin D due to malabsorption, leading to rickets, ostopenia and osteoporosis. Reversal of symptoms is observed on gluten withdrawal from the diet.
- **Lactose Intolerance:** Due to flattening of the mucosal villi, the lactase enzyme cannot be produced leading to lactose intolerance. Once the gluten free diet is initiated, the lactase enzyme is reversed and the child is able to tolerate lactose based products.
- **Cancer:** Studies have proven that long standing untreated CD leads to an increased risk of gastrointestinal cancer like lymphoma, but such incidences are very rare.
- **Neurological and Psychiatric complications:** Symptoms of depression, neuropathy, balance disorders, seizures and severe headaches are known to be associated with consequences of untreated CD.
- **Short Stature:** malabsorption in celiac who continue to include gluten in their diets can lead to deprivation of the essential nutrients which can result in stunted growth and short stature.
- **Miscarriages and Congenital Malformations of the Fetus:** Undiagnosed pregnant women who are unaware of their celiac status, not on GFD, have a risk of neural tube defect, miscarriages or congenital malformation.

- **Milk Protein Enteropathy:** Milk protein allergy has also been reported in celiac but are known to resolve by age of 2 years.[22]
- **Autoimmune Disease:** Conditions like liver abnormalities with raised aminotransferase levels, hepatic dysfunction, diabetes mellitus, IgA deficiency, cystic fibrosis and thyroid diseases have been associated with prolonged untreated or inadequately treated gluten enteropathy.

CELIAC CRISIS

This is a condition manifested by profuse watery diarrhea, dehydration and shock mostly occurring during a gluten challenge or if during the course of GFD, the child suddenly starts gluten either inadverdently or on the sly. This condition is reversible if treated promptly.[1]

RECIPES FOR GLUTEN FREE DIET

Gram Laddoo

Green gram.................................... 20 g
Whole corn seeds .... 20 g
Groundnuts.................................... 8 g
Sugar/Jaggery................................. 20 g

- Roast corn whole, green gram and groundnuts and grind them to a powder
- Make jaggery syrup, add the flour mixture
- Mix well and make into balls.

Chidwa Barfi

Pressed rice .... 25 g
Roasted groundnut .... 20 g
Jaggery .... 25 g

- Roast the pressed rice and mix with groundnuts
- Add the pressed rice and nuts and mix quickly
- Spread the above mixture on a greased plate and cut into pieces immediately.
- This recipe is extensively used in special nutrition program in Andhra Pradesh.[23]

Chidwa Laddoo

Chidwa .... 35 g
Roasted groundnuts........................ 20 g
Roasted Bengal gram .... 25 g
Sugar/Jaggery................................. 25 g

- Powder chidwa, roasted bengal gram dal, groundnuts and sugar and mix the powders.
- Add hot water to make the mixture soft in consistency and make into laddoos.

Dosa

Green gram dal (washed)................ 25 g
Black gram dal (washed) .... 25 g
Soyabean... 25 g
Salt .... to taste
Oil .... 3 tsp
Water... 3-4 tsps

- Soak all thc three dals separately overnight
- Remove skin from soyabean by rubbing with hands
- Mix greengram dal, black gram dal, soyabeans and grind to paste
- Add water and prepare the batter. Stir the batter well and keep aside covered for 4 hours to ferment
- Add salt and mix thoroughly
- Grease the pan, heat and pour on to it
- Cook lightly till golden brown using oil on both sides.

Sago Kheer

Sago.. 100 g
Sugar .... 30 g
Grated coconut............................... 10 g
Food colour .... 1 drop
Water .... for cooking

- Cook sago and sugar in water till soft and the mixture thickens
- Add color and cook till soft and the mixture binds
- Make into balls and dust with grated coconut.

Rice Pura

Rice powder/flour............................ 50 g
Salt .... to taste
Curd... 20 g
Oil .... for frying

- Mix rice powder, curd and salt to make a smooth batter
- Heat the pan and spreadout a little batter to form a thin pura
- Fry lightly on both sides till done.

Idli

Rice .... 75 g
Black gram dal (washed) .... 25 g
Salt .... to taste

- Soak rice and moong dal separately for 5-6 hours
- Grind both separately and mix together
- Add salt and keep aside overnight, covered, to allow to ferment
- Pour ladel full of mixture on the compartmental sytand which are slightly greased
- Place the stand into a pressure cooker filled with water to form steam
- Cover the pressure cooker and remove the done idlis on to a plate.

Note: The same batter can be used to make dosa by making it into a pouring consistency and spreading it on a pan to shallow fry on both sides.

SAMPLE MENU FOR GLUTEN FREE DIET

Breakfast	Maize roti/ 1-2
	Idli/dosa...................................1-2
	Egg ....1 (optional)
	Curd/Milk.................................200 ml
Mid Morning	Poha/Dhokla/Besan pura/Fruit
Lunch	Rice ....2 servings
	Dal..1 serving
	Vegetable..................................1 serving
	Curd..100 g
	Salad
Evening	Soya porridge/sago kheer/rice kheer (using milk-200 ml)
Dinner	Missi roti/rice ....1-2/50-75 g
	Paneer/chicken/dal ....30 g/100 g/serving
Bed time	Milk..150 ml

REFERENCES

1. Dicke WK. Celiakeie:een onderzoek naar de nadelige involved van sommige graanoorte op de ligder aan coeliake. M.D. thesis, Utrecht and Transactions of the 6th International Congress of Pediatrics, 1950; pp.117, Zurich.

2. Pauley LW. Observation on the etiology of idiopathic steatorrhea. Br Med J 1954;2:1318-20.
3. Walia BNS, Sidhu JK, Ghai OP. Celiac Disease in North Indian children. Br Med J 1966;2:1233-4.
4. Walker-Smith JA. Celiac disease, *In*: Diseases of the Small Intestine in Childhood, 2nd Ed (ed. Walker-Smith JA). London: Pitman Medical 1979.
5. Myollete M, Egan Mitchelle B, Fottrell PF, et al. Incidence of celiac disease in the west of Ireland. Br Med J 1973;1:703-5.
6. Thapa BR. Celiac Disese: Indian experience. In: Nutrition in Children, Developing Countries Concerns. 1994, Sachdev HPS and Chaudhary P (Eds). Dept. of Pediatrics, Maulana Azad Medical College, New Delhi.
7. Rubin CE, Brandborg LL, Flick AL, et al. Biopsy studies on the pathogenesis of celiac sprue. In: Intestinal Biopsy (ed. Wolstenholme GEW and Cameron MP) 1962;pp67, Edinburgh: Churchill Livingstone.
8. WHO Proposed draft standard for gluten free products. Codex Alimentarius Commission ALINORM 79/26 Appendix 2 Step 8, 1979;pp19-20.
9. Walker-Smith LA. Celiac disease. In: Diseases of the Small Intestine in Childhood, 3rd ed, London, Butterworths, 1988;88-143.
10. Tria JS. Celiac disease. In: Gastrointestinal Disease; Pathophysiology, Diagnosis and Management, 5th ed. Sleisenger M, Fordtran JS (Eds) Phildelphia, WB Saunders Company, 193;1078-96.
11. Branski D, Fasano A, Trancone R. Latest Developments in the pathogenesis and treatment of celiac disease. J Pediatr 2006;149:295-300.
12. Cook DM, Evans N, Lloyd A, Strwart JS. Normal serum and red cell folate levels in a child with celiac disease. Lancet 1970;1, 571-2.
13. Meeuwisse GW. Round Table discussion. Diagnostic criteria for celiac disease. Acta Pediatr Scand 1970;59:461-68.
14. Sahni A, Thapa BR, Malik AK, Meehta S. Jujunal mucosal histology. Critical appraisal of criteria for diagnosis of CD. Abstracts. 25th Annual Conference of IA, Jodhpur 24-28 Oct,198.
15. Hill ID, Bhatnagar S, Cameron DJS, De RS Maki M, Russel GJ, Trancone R. Celiac Disease: Working Group Repot of the First World Congress of pediatric Gastroenterology, Hepatology and Nutrition. J Pediatr Gastroenterol Nutr 2002; 35: Supplement 2:S78-88.
16. Norris J Barrriga K, Klingensmith G, et al. Timing of initial cereal exposure in infancy and risk of islet autoimmunity. JAMA 2003;290:1713-2.
17. Weile B, Cavell B, Nivenius K, et al. Striking differences in the incidence of childhood celiac disease between Denmark and Sweden: A possible explanation. J Pediatr Gastroenterol Nutr 1995;21:64-8.
18. Carlson A, Agardh D, Borulf S, et al. Prevalence of celiac disease: Before and after a national change in feeding recommendations. Scand J Gastroenterol 2006;41:533-5.

19. Ivarsson A, Hernell O, Stenlud H, et al. Breast feeding protects against celiac disease. Am J Clin Nutr 2002;75:914-21.
20. Akobeng AK, Ramanan AV, Buvhan I, Heller RF. Effect of breastfeeding on risk of CD: A systematic review and meta analysis of observational studies. Arch Dis child 2006;91:39-43.
21. National Institute of Health. Consensus Development Conference Statement. June 28-30,2004,see website About.com:http://consensus.nik.gov/2004,celiac disease 118 html.htm.
22. Watt J, Pincott JR, harris JT. Combined cow's milk protein and gluten induced enteropathy: commonor rare? Gut 24, 1983;165-70.
23. National Institute of nutrition, ICMR, Hyderabad, India (1977), Low Cost Nutritious Supplements.

Chapter 6 Diet in Inflammatory Bowel Disease

Inflammatory bowel disease (IBD) comprises two main entities:

- Crohn's disease (CD)
- Ulverative colitis (UC)

The characteristic features of inflammatory bowel disease are weight loss and nutritional deficiencies. Crohn's disease can involve any part of the gastrointestinal tract (GIT), while ulcerative colitis is mostly confined to the colon with minimal involvement of the terminal ileum.[1]

Both CD and UC may present with overlapping signs and symptoms like diarrhea, GI bleed, protein loss, abdominal pain, weight loss, anemia and growth failure. Abdominal pain accounts for almost 72 percent of IBD diarrhea and weight loss presents in about 56 percent and 58 percent of the children while only 25 percent of the cases may present with growth failure. As CD involves mainly the terminal ileum, it was described as ileitis. But recent reports also give evidence of Crohn's involving the gastroduodenal section in about 50 percent of the cases and about 20 percent involving the jejunum.[2]

INCIDENCE

IBD is now emerging as a major challenge for pediatricians, especially so, in the industrialized countries and it is believed that childhood IBD accounts for about 30 percent of the total cases reported. The reason for this has been attributed to partly certain environmental factors like hygiene, diet, breastfeeding, smoking (antenatal period), oral contraceptive pills and infectious agents like mumps, measles, etc.[3]

In the Pediatric Inflammatory Bowel disease Clinic at St. Bartholomew's Hospital from 1978-1995, and then from 1995-99 at the Free Hospital at London, there were reported to be about 30-40 new children referred each year. In the UK, estimates put the incidence of CD per 100,000 children as 10.7, while in Japan it has been indicated to be only 0.6 percent.[4]

Although, IBD has extensively been reported from the Western countries, the incidence is not uncommon in India also. Estimates from Indian observations report about 5 percent of the total admissions for colonic disorders as UC in children.[5] Similar observations have been reported from other parts of India.[6,7] In fact there seems to be an increasing trend mainly for CD in childhood. A recent study from Chennai reported the clinical manifestations of CD in children and adolescents. The youngest child reported from South India is 4 years and 6 months who presented unusually with palatal ulcer.[8]

According to an epidemiological review by Sood from North India,[9] there is convincing evidence of rising trend of IBD in Asian countries and India probably heads the list, sadly catching-up with the West. In his words, 'ulcerative colitis is already here and we have to brace ourselves to face the onslaught of Crohn's disease in coming years.' The same may hold true in the case of pediatric age group too.

AGE OF ONSET OF INFLAMMATORY BOWEL DISEASE

Varied reports on age of onset of IBD in children are available but it is observed that children less than 5 years of age comprise about 4 percent of the pediatric Crohn's disease, while the modern age of presentation of CD is 7.9 years.[10] Though IBD can manifest at any age, it is rarely seen in infancy. Only1 percent of IBD children are diagnosed before one year of age.[11] Armitage observed an association of CD with affluence. It was suggested that this may be due to low level/delayed exposure to common childhood infectious agents due to improved domestic hygiene resulting in altered immune response in genetically susceptible host the so called 'hygiene hypothesis'.[12]

Recent data from the British Isles have shown that significantly greater proportion of children of Asian origin feature among under 5 with IBD (25 percent vs 6 percent) with a relative risk of 3:9.[2] The first national prospective survey of childhood IBD from the British Isles documented an incidence of 5.2/100,000 children and less than 16 years per year.[13] It is believed that the incidence increases steadily with age during childhood and adolescence peaking at about 14 years of age. Unlike in adults pediatric onset CD has clear male preponderance. In the UK study, 62 percent of pediatric CD in a cohort of 379 children were males.[2]

PATHOGENESIS

As mentioned earlier Crohn's disease and ulcerative colitis both have many features in common like diarrhea, GI bleed, abdominal pain, weight loss, anemia and a number of nutritional deficiencies. Approximately 30 percent of children with CD are have growth failure and children with

CD are three times as likely to have permanent growth stunting than are patients with UC.[14]

The onset is often insidious and may remain undiagnosed for long. By the time the diagnosis is pinpointed, the child has possibly lost his precious years of growth resulting in considerable failure to thrive due to inadequate intake, besides nutritional loses associated with the disease. At times extraintestinal manifestations may be observed which could comprise 25-30 percent of children with IBD and these may remain undiagnosed for many years. Recurrent apthous ulcers is the most common manifestation of IBD and a frequent finding in Crohn's disease.[15,16] Other disease specific manifestations include the oral cavity like mucosal tags, lip swelling, fissures, buccal swelling or cobble stoning, deep linear ulcerations and localised mucogingivitis[17] Unusual manifestations like just oral lesions in the form of a palatal ulcer has been reported without the presence of any other reported symptoms in a child from South India who was perhaps the youngest reported from India.[18]

NUTRITIONAL IMPLICATIONS OF IBD IN CHILDREN

The range of nutritional problems developing in IBD as given in Table 6.1 may have the following implications.[19]

a. Immunologic impairment and increased incidence of infection.
b. Poor wound and fistula healing.
c. Decreased tolerance to blood loss.
d. Increased morbidity and mortality following surgical intervention.

NUTRITIONAL MANAGEMENT OF IBD

For management of IBD it is important to know what are the factors which predispose to malnutrition in such children. Table 6.2 gives a brief picture of the possible causes:

GOALS OF MANAGEMENT OF CROHN'S DISEASE AND ULCERATIVE COLITIS

1. To induce remission.
2. To maintain remission.
3. To maintain optimal growth and development.
4. To optimize nutritional support and prevent deficiency state.

Crohn's Disease

As mentioned earlier, Crohn's disease is more prevalent in the pediatric age group and therefore the main implication in them is growth failure

Table 6.1: Frequency of nutritional deficiencies reported in patients with IBD

Nutritional Deficiencies	*Percentage*
Weight loss	65-75
Growth Retardation	15-30
Hypoalbumenimia	25-80
Anemia	60-80
Iron Deficiency	48
Vitamin B_{12}	36-54
Calcium Deficiency	13
Magnesium deficiency	14-33
Potassium deficiency	6-20
Vitamin A deficiency	11
Vitamin C deficiency	*
Vitamin D deficiency	75
Vitamin K deficiency	40-50
Copper deficiency	*
Vitamin E deficiency	*
Metabolic bone disease	*

*Reported but prevalence not described.

Table 6.2: Causative factors of malnutrition in IBD

Inadequate Intake
Anorexia, altered taste
Abdominal pain, diarrhea, nausea, vomiting
Restrictive diet
Malabsorption
Diminished digestive function secondary to decreased bile salts
Diminished absorptive surface area secondary to extensive disease and/or previous bowel resection
Drug induced malabsorption, e.g steroid/calcium
Increased GI losses
Protein losing enteropathy
GI bleed
Electrolyte and mineral loss
Increased Nutritional Requirements
Fever, fistula, infection
Repletion of body stores

due to the reasons cited in Table 6.2. It has been demonstrated that introduction of nutritional repletion reverses growth failure along with induction of remission.[20,21] Nutritional support for children with Crohn's disease involves either enteral in the form of elemental diet or parenteral nutrition. At times a combination of the two may also be used. Elemental diets have been used with success in most centers.

Elemental Diets

Elemental diets can be described as a chemically defined diet with amino acids or short chain peptides as the protein source along with short chain carbohydrates and added fat, minerals and vitamins. It is observed that almost 50-60 percent of the children with CD when treated with enteral nutrition in clinical trials achieve clinical remission.[22] It has been recommended that enteral nutrition should be the sole source of nutrition as offering regular food may compromise efficiency,[23] since the child tends to get full sooner and thereby may not tolerate the formulated feed. However, oral sips of water or clear fluids may be allowed. Nasogastric feeding tubes have been recommended for night feeding to compensate any deficit intake during day time. Enteral nutrition is thought to bring about some extensive changes within the gut, some of them being:

- Bowel rest
- Reduction in antigenic load
- Low resilience diet
- Correction of nutritional deficit
- Alteration of gut flora

The enteral nutrition formula should be such that it provides 100 percent of the child's estimated requirements for energy and proteins. The volume should be increased gradually as per individual tolerance. Polymeric peptide based and amino acid based diets have also been used to treat active CD, and if a child can drink orally, a polymeric liquid diet can be encouraged due to its greater palatability.

The duration of exclusive enteral feeding has been recommended to continue for a minimum of 4 weeks or longer if the child has not attained the desired weight and height. Gradual introduction of semisolids to solids is done, preferably with a low fiber diet as shown in Table 6.3.

Observations have pointed out that almost 60-70 percent of the patients experience a relapse within 1 year of stopping enteral nutrition, therefore two nutritional strategies have been considered to maintain remission:

1. Cyclical exclusive enteral nutrition in which nocturnal feeding is continued without regular food, once in 4 months.[24]
2. Supplementary enteral nutrition in which nocturnal nasogastrofeeding is continued 4-5 times weekly as a supplement to unrestricted daytime diet.[25]

The success of the therapy is marked by normal and catch-up linear growth of children treated for CD. If a child does not show linear growth velocity despite weight gain, it is an indicator that the inflamed intestine has not healed completely and might call for other methods

Table 6.3: Dietary regimen for introduction of solid foods

Days of introduction	*Type of foods*	*Example*
1-4	Low fiber cereals	White bread, rice, biscuits plain, cereal pulse (khichdi)
5-9	Pulses washed/fish/eggs	Washed dals, fish (low fat), eggs chicken tender, tofu
10-14	Low fiber vegetables	Raw fruits without skin, membrane Fruits tender cooked vegetable without skin seeds, plain soup, noodles
15-17	Low fat dairy products	Toned/skimmed milk yogurt cottage cheese
18	Regular diet as per tolerance	Increase fat and fiber gradually

of treatment. Inappropriate use of corticosteroids are known to impede catch-up height velocity due to the contributory growth inhibiting effects of proinflammatory cytokines produced by the inflamed intestine.

NUTRITIONAL DEFICIENCIES

Most of the children with CD suffer from multiple vitamin and mineral deficiencies due to the malabsorptive state of the gut, poor intake and intestinal losses some of which are discussed as under:

Vitamins and minerals: Most Indian children on vegetarian diets may not be able to get the folic acid sources like animal foods and hence supplements need to be provided. Even if they are nonvegetarians, due to poor absorption it may be deficient in them. Use of certain medications like sulfasalazine inhibit folic acid absorption too. And hence supplementing this becomes essential.

Other nutrients like vitamins B_{12}, magnesium and vitamin E are also known to be deficient in them which need supplementation (Table 6.4). Foods like banana and potatoes are good sources of magnesium and including them in the diet of such children can be beneficial. But large doses of oral supplements may exert a laxative effect and hence needs to be given inmoderation or monitored as per requirement.

Iron, calcium and vitamin D may also be deficient in children with IBD (Crohn's disease). Iron can interfere with calcium if taken together and may also be a gastric irritant, therefore iron supplements need to be appropriately selected and advised. Encouraging foods rich in iron like green leafy vegetables, banana and cooking in iron pans can enhance the iron content of diets of such children. Use of ascorbic acid in food in the form of lemon or other citrus fruits if tolerated can enhance absorption of iron.

Table 6.4: Vitamin and mineral supplements for children with IBD

Nutrients	*Dose*
Multivitamin with mineral	1 tab. daily
Iron	4-6 mg/Kg in 3 divided doses
Folate (for sulfasalazine therapy)	1 mg/d
Vitamin B_{12}	1 mg I q 3 months
Calcium	1200 mg
Zinc	50-100 mg
Magnesium	200-400 mg

Source: A.M. Davis etal. Pediatric Gastroenterintestinal Disorders, In: The ASPEN Nutrition Support Practice Manual. R. Meeritt ed. pp27:12-13.

Small frequent feeding would be a better way to feed children and the preparations can be formulated such that the caloric density of the feeds can be enhanced. Larger bolus feeds tend to put off children from eating besides triggering abdominal pain and bloating, therefore best avoided.

Fluid requirements also need to be kept in mind to avoid dehydration in the presence of frequent stooling.

Probiotics: The role of probiotics in minimizing gastrointestinal symptoms in children with IBD has been considered by some authors. Usually the lactobacillus or the acidophilus forms available in capsule form can perhaps help normalize intestinal function by restoring a healthy balance. Children who are intolerant to milk, may benefit by curd which is a natural probiotic. The role of prebiotics like psyllium has also been suggested in the healing process.

Marine food: The use of fish oil and flaxseed oil has been considered by various authors in patients with IBD. Fish oil therapy in the form of enteric coated capsules is known to be effective in preventing relapses in patients with Crohn's disease in remission.[26] Patients with ulcerative colitis too have been shown to demonstrate positive results by use of fish oil and supplements. It was speculated that the EPA in the fish oil interferes with the symptoms of the highly inflammatory leukotriene B4 in the lining of the colon and that effect accounts for the improvement.[27] It was suggested that fish oil may work by reducing existing inflammation but that it may not necessarily be effective in preventing inflammation. Further research needs to confirm these observations.

Ulcerative Colitis (UC)

In UC the aim is to maintain remission as in case of CD. The principle of nutritional management is same as that applied in case of CD where growth failure along with the nutritional deficiencies coexists. Corticosteroids are usually recommended in children having extensive involvement of the colon. Fluid and electrolyte needs to be balanced along with blood and albumin transfusion if excess blood loss occurs. Most of the children may require surgery in which case nutritional rehabilitation (with appropriate nutrients) is an important component of the treatment.

Summary of Dietary Support for IBD in Children

- Maintain hydration of the patient by ensuring a good fluid intake which will also prevent constipation
- A high fiber diet when child is in remission
- During a flare up, limit fiber in the diet as also a low residue diet should be encouraged. This gives rest to the bowels and minimize symptoms
- Avoid lactose containing foods (milk and other milk concentrated foods)
- Small frequent feeding should be encouraged rather than 2-3 bolus feeds
- The diet should be high in protein and calories. Fats should be moderate and MCT (medium chain triglycerides) might be a good option as these are better tolerated as compared to the polyunsaturated or saturated fats. Coconut oil is an example of MCT which can be used as a cooking medium. Fried foods or other high fat foods need to be avoided
- Tea and coffee should be avoided as there can irritate the bowel and exacerbate symptoms
- Restrict gas producing foods like cabbage, cauliflower, sprouts and gram, dried peas, onions pepper and carbonated drinks
- Use of fish and fish oil and flaxseeds can be beneficial for such patients due to their high omega 3 contents which exert an antiinflammatory effect
- Probiotics especially with live culture like curd can also prove beneficial for such patients.

Sample Menu for Children with IBD

Early Morning	Water	1-2 glasses
Breakfast	Cereal	1 serving (Suji/dalia sewain)
	Curd	1 serving
	Egg-(optional)	1 serving
Mid Morning	Brown bread/Cereal (poha/dalia, etc.)	
	Buttermilk (if tolerated)/Veg. soup	

Lunch	Cereal (Rice/Chapatti)
	Pulses (washed)................1 serving
	Soft green vegetables ....1 serving
	Curd (if tolerated).............1 serving
Evening	Herbal tea
	Biscuits/Rusk....................1-2
Dinner	Cereal (as for lunch)
	Pulse/Chicken/Fish...........1 serving
	Soft Vegetables.................1 serving
	Salad (if in remission) ....as desired

REFERENCES

1. Motil KJ, Grand RJ. Inflammatory Bowel disease. In: Walker WA, Watkins JB, (Eds). Nutrition in Pediatrics: Basic science and Clinical Applications. Hamilton, Ontario; BC Decka; 1997;516.
2. Saweczenko A, Sandhu BK. Presenting features of IBD in Great Britain and Ireland. Arch Dis Child 2003; 88: 995-1000.
3. Buller H, Chin S, Kirschnen B, Kohn J, et al. Inflammatory Bowel Disease I children and adolescents: Working Group Report of First World Congress of Pediatric Gastroenterology Hepatology and Nutrition, J Pediatr Gastroenterol Nutr 2002;35: (Suppl 2) S 151-58.
4. Robert B Heuschkel, John A Walker Smith, Enteral Nutrition in IBD of Childhood. J Enter Parenteral Nutr 1999;23;5:529-532.
5. Mehta S. Inflammatory Bowel Diseases in Children: Indian perspective. Ind J Pediatr 1999;587-88.
6. R.Ganesh, N Singh, S ezhilarasis, Sarala Rajajee and Malathi Sathiyasekaran. Crohn's disease presenting as Palatal Ulcer. Ind J Pediatr 2006;73(3):229-331.
7. Vikrant Khana, Abhinav Sharma, Harsh Deep Sahni, Ujjal Poddar, S.K. yachha. Inflammatory Bowel Disease: Clinical Spectrum in North India. Prdgastro 2005- Conference abstracts, Pediatric on Call, http://www.pediatric on call.com/for doctor/conference_abstracts.
8. Malathi S, Bhaskar Raju B, Shivbalan So, Rajarajan K. Pediatric Crohn's Disease in South India. Indian Pediatrics, 2005;42:459-463.
9. Sood A, Midha V. Epidemiology of bowel disease in Asia. Indian J Gastroenterol 2007; 26:285-9.
10. Baldaasson RN, Piccoli DA. Inflammatory bowel disease in pediatric and adolescent patients. Gastroenterol Clin N Am 1999;28:445-55.
11. Armitage EL, Alhdous MC, Anderson N, Drummond HE , Ghosh S, et al. Incidence of juvenile onset of Crohn's disease in Scotland: Association with Northern latitude and affluence. Gastroenetrology 2004; 127:1051-57.
12. Montogomery SM, Pounder RE, Wakefield AJ. Infant mortality and the incidence of inflammatory bowel disease. Lancet 1997;349: 427-73.

13. Sawczenko A, Sandhu BK, Logan RF, Jenkins H, et al. Prospective survey of childhood inflammatory disease. Lancet 2001;357:1093-94.
14. Motil KJ, Grand RJ. Inflammatory bowel disease. In: Basic Sciences and Clinical Applications. Walker WA, Watkins JB (Eds) Hamilton, Ontario: BC Decker; 1997;516.
15. Walker Smith JA. Disease of the Small Intestine in Childhood. 2nd Ed. London Pitman Meical, 1979.
16. Pittock S, Drumm B, Fleming P, Mc Dermott, et al. The oral cavity in Crohn's disease. J Ped iatr 2002;138(5):767-71.
17. Ganesh R, Suresh N, Ezhilarari S, Rajajee Sarala, Sathyasekaran M. Crohn's Disease presenting as palatal ulcer. Ind J Ped, 2006;73;3:229-31.
18. Melissa F, Perkell, John H. Seashore. Nutrition and IBD. Gastroenterology Clinics of North America 1989;18; 3:567-77.
19. Melissa F, Perkell, John H. Seashore. Nutrition and Inflammatory Bowel Disease, Gastroenterology Clinics of North America 1989;18;3:567-77.
20. Kirschner BS, Klich JR, Kalman SS, De Favaro MV, Rosenberg IH. Reversal of growth retardation in Crohn's disease with therapy emphasizing oral nutrition restitution. Gastroenterology 1981;80,10-15.
21. O'Moran CA, Segal AW, Levi AJ. Elemental diets in the treatment of acute Crohn's disease: A controlled study. Gut 23, 891.
22. Griffiths AM, Ohlsson A, Sherman PM, Sutherland LR, Metaanalysis of enteral nutrition as a primary treatment of active Crohn's disease. Gastroenetrology 1995;108:1056-67.
23. Johnson T, Mac Donald S, Hill SM, et al. Treatment of active Crohn's disease in children using partial enteral nutrition with liquid formula: A randomized control trial. Gut 2006;55:356-61.
24. Belli DC, Seidman E, Bouthillier F, et al. Chronic intermittent diet improves growth failure in children with Crohn's disease. Gastroenterology 1988;94:603-10.
25. Wilschanski M, Sherman P, Pencharz P, et al. Supplementary enteral nutrition maintains remission in pediatric Crohn's Disease Gut 1996;38:543-48.
26. Belluzz IA, Brignola C, Campieri M, et al. Effects of an enteric coated fish oil preparation on relapses in Crohn's disease. The N Eng J Med 1996, Vol 334, No.24, June 13, 1996;1557-60.
27. Salomon Pete, et al. The treatment of ulcerative colitis with fish oil in n-3 omega fatty acid: An open trial. J Clin Gastroenterol 1990;12; 2: 157-61.

Chapter 7 Nutritional Support in Cystic Fibrosis

Cystic fibrosis (CF) is the most common autosomal recessive disorder found predominantly in the Caucasian population with an incidence of 1:25000 live births[1] and 1 in 25 of the population are carriers.

The disease involves widespread dysfunction of the exocrine glands with disturbances in the ion and fluid movement resulting in abnormally thick and dehydrated secretions. There are multiorgan lesions including:

- Chronic obstructive lung disease with predominant airway obstruction and recurrent, persistent infection
- Exocrine pancreatic insufficiency with steatorrhea
- Intestinal obstruction in neonates and older patients
- Abnormally high levels of sodium chloride sweat, resulting from the failure of salt reabsorption in sweat gland ducts.

The basic defect in CF is a mutational change in the gene for chloride conductance channel called cystic fibrosis transmembrane conductance regulator (CFTR). Failure of chloride conductance by epithelial cells leads to dehydration of secretions that are too vivid and difficult to clear.

The prevalence of genetic mutation varies from one population to the other the commonest one being the delta 508 which constitutes almost 70 percent of the total cases. The frequency of this mutation among Asians migrated to U.K. is almost less than 50 percent. In view of these figures, CF cannot be considered rare among Indians. The diagnosis is usually delayed due to late suspicion. These patients are mostly treated as tuberculosis, pneumonia and acute exacerbations are labeled as 'bronchopneumonia'. Lack of diagnostic facilities especially a standardized sweat test could be one reason why so few patients have been reported so far.[2]

Gastrointestinal (GI) involvement is present in 85-90 percent of all cases and symptoms generally appear before age of 2 years but may remain undiagnosed for many years.

CLINICAL PRESENTATION

Children diagnosed with CF may present with features associated with different organs but the most commonly seen are those involving the respiratory and the GI functions (Table 7.1).

Pancreatic Insufficiency

A child usually appears normal in size at birth. There is progressive destruction of exocrine pancreas, leading to impaired intraluminal hydrolysis of dietary lipids and proteins. By age of 2 months the child gradually begins to show signs of protein energy malnutrition with or without diarrhea.[3] GI involvement is present in 85-95 percent of all cases. Due to the pancreatic damage involved, the secretion of digestive enzymes and bicarbonate is affected, resulting in malabsorption of fat, proteins, nitrogen, bile, fat soluble vitamins and B_{12}. According to estimates, in 90 percent of the patients, the enzyme secretion is absent making them pancreatic enzyme dependent. In the rest 10 percent of

Table 7.1: Clinical features of cystic fibrosis

Intestines	Abdominal pain Rectal prolapsed Distal intestinal obstruction Steatorrhea/Diarrhea Abdominal distension Failure to thrive Gastrocolic reflux
Pancreas	Pancreatic failure Pancreatitis Glucose intolerance Diabetes mellitus
Gallbladder	Cholecystitis Cholelithiasis Obstructive jaundice
Lungs	Recurrent respiratory infections Asthma Nasal polyps Bronchiectasis Hyperventilation Clubbing of fingers Hemoptysis Pneumothorax
Others	Delayed puberty Salt depletion Male sterility Arthritis Fat soluble deficiencies

the patients, the enzyme secretions are present but in minimal amounts adequate for digestion and absorption of nutrients without the need for enzyme supplementation.

Due to the defect in absorption of nutrients, growth failure is most frequently encountered among these children, ultimately resulting in delayed puberty.

Chronic Respiratory Involvement

The lungs are normal at birth, but may get affected within a few weeks of life. There are abnormal secretions resulting in mucoid production which cause obstruction in the small airways, with secondary infection which is progressive and destructive. The child has persistent cough productive of purulent sputum.

Gastroesophageal Reflux (GER)

GER is a common feature observed among some patients with CF which could be due to inappropriate reaction of the gastroesophageal sphincter. Though it is more frequent among younger age group, the incidence decreases with age.

Growth Failure

The next common problem among children with CF is chronic malnutrition with significant weight loss and failure to thrive. Malnutrition is generally an associated feature observed among most children with CF, which can be prevented or corrected with adequate nutritional measures.

CAUSES OF MALNUTRITION

Nutrition: A Risk Factor

Early detection of nutritional risk is necessary in order to intervene at a time when a proactive approach can make a positive impact on the outcome.[4] Studies have demonstrated that low weight if not corrected can itself pose an independent risk factor of survival.[5]

There is a set criteria defined by the Clinical Practice Guidelines for Cystic Fibrosis Foundation for classifying nutritional status in patients with cystic fibrosis[6] which has been laid down by the Metropolitan Life Insurance company in the USA[7] as presented in Table 7.2.

Nutritional problems in CF are determined by 3 factors:

- Energy losses
- Increased energy expenditure
- Decreased energy intake.

Table 7.2: Definition of nutritional status in patients with cystic fibrosis

Age group	*At risk*	*Nutritional failure*
0-2 years	Weight for length 10-15 percent	Height percentile <5% OR Weight for length <10% OR IBW <90%
2-20 years	BMI percentile 10th-25th	BMI percentile <10% OR IBW(<90%)
Adults	BMI 19-20	BMI <19 OR Percent IBW<90%

Ref. 6

Energy Losses

There are significant energy losses due to presence of malabsorption of proteins and fats. It has been estimated that stool energy losses account for 11 percent of gross energy intake in CF patients, three times higher than normal.[8] Losses also may occur through vomiting following bouts of cough or gastroesophageal reflux which is commonly seen in such children, Nitrogen losses may occur through sputum (rich in amino acids) during severe acute pulmonary exacerbations.

Increased Energy Expenditure

Abnormal pulmonary mechanisms may increase the resting energy expenditure. Continuous injury to the lungs causing airway obstruction can be associated with increased oxygen cost and breathing.[9]

Low Energy Intake

It is generally seen that the energy intake of most children with CF remains very low resulting in suboptimal growth pattern. This low intake could be due to several factors like:

- Anorexia
- Chronic respiratory infections and other complications of CF like abdominal pain, GER, resulting in vomiting and pain.
- Behavior feeding problems in school and preschool children encountered in even normal children.
- Depression
- Eating disorders in adolescents
- Dislike of high energy foods
- Poverty, ignorance and food fads.

GOALS OF NUTRITIONAL MANAGEMENT

The three main objectives of nutritional management are:

1. To achieve optimal nutritional status.
2. To achieve normal growth and development.

3. To maintain normal feeding behavior.

   The approach to achieve these goals is 2 pronged:

- Nutritional support
- Pancreatic enzyme supplementation (PES).

Nutritional Support

Energy

The energy requirements of patients with CF are estimated to be around 120-150 percent of the recommended daily allowances (RDA) for age and sex. But usually such patients are unable to meet these standards in the Indian population. As they are already caloric deficit, initially they should be to bring their intake levels to the RDA and then gradually further build up to meet the estimated requirements. The presence of respiratory infections, activity and nutritional status makes it difficult to follow a set universal pattern. The best way to monitor the intake is by monitoring their growth velocity. A useful guideline to follow is to assess the existing energy intake and increase this value by a further 20-30 percent if weight gain or growth is poor.

Proteins

Protein requirements should be increased to compensate for excessive loss of nitrogen in the stools and sputum and increased protein turnover in malnourished children. About 150-200 percent of RDA can be provided by proteins.

Fats

It is widely accepted that fat being the most concentrated source of energy, should be encouraged. Most often it is observed that parents tend to restrict fat content of the diets of their children with CF in view of increased losses in stools, thinking that it will not be digested. This myth needs to be discouraged and parents should be explained the importance of fat sources in the diet. The malabsorption of fats can be dealt with supplementation of pancreatic enzymes as will be discussed further in this chapter. The role of medium chain triglycerides to be substituted for other oils is controversial and not widely accepted, with the view that it may result in deficiency of essential fatty acids and indirectly increase energy requirements as it needs more oxygen than carbohydrates to be oxidized in the liver.[10]

Carbohydrates

About 40-50 percent of the energy intake should be provided by carbohydrate sources which are well tolerated. High starch foods like bread, potatoes and pasta as well as simple sugars can be used liberally in the diet of such children. Table 7.3 summarizes the recommendations for nutrient intakes in children with CF.[11,12,13]

FEEDING OF INFANTS

Breast Milk

Breastfeeds being high in lipase content in combination with pancreatic enzymes. The advantages of doing so have been highlighted as follows:[14,15]

- It contains long chain fatty acids.
- It provides immunological protection against infections
- It contains taurine
- It contains optimal essential amino acids.
- It is psychologically better for the mother.

However, as mentioned earlier, due to the increased energy losses in them, breast milk alone may not be adequate to meet their requirement and hence formula feeds will have to be supplemented. Calorie dense commercial supplements can be incorporated along with formula milk.

For children intolerant to cow's milk or are lactose intolerant, hydrolysed protein formulae are good substitutes. To meet the enhanced caloric requirements of babies with CF in enzyme therapy, extra fats can be used. The deficiency of essential fatty acids (EFA) can be made up with vegetable oils rather than butter.

Table 7.3: Recommendations for Nutritional Management in Cystic Fibrosis

Protein	120 percent of RDA
Energy	Variable depending on disease status but should average at least 115 percent of RDA
Fats	40 percent of total energy as LCT and 3-5 percent as EFA
Micronutrients	Vitamin A............... 5000-10,000 IU/d*
	Vitamin D............... 400-800 IU/d**
	Vitamin E............... Infants-50 mg
	Children.................. 100 mg
	Adolescents........... 200 mg

*If serum levels normal, may not require supplements.
**Regular exposure to sunlight is adequate in most warm climates.

Feeding of Older Children

As for normal children, by one year of age the child should be fed from the 'family pot', but ensuring to incorporate the feeds such that the enhanced requirements are met with small frequent feeding of high density foods. This could be achieved by 5-6 small but frequent thickened or dense feeds. A bed time snack is a good idea for tiding over the long gap at night time. To ensure adequate intake, regular growth monitoring is the best and simplest way which even parents can record. A suboptimal weight gain or static weight over a prolonged period of time is an indicator of inadequate intake or enzyme dosage. With normal weight gain, the use of supplements (commercial) can be avoided. Even if offered, it should not replace the meals. Standard age related recommendations for the calorie contribution from supplements to the diet of a patient with CF have been laid down as follows:[16]

1-2 years.......... 200 cals/d
3-5 years.......... 400 cals/d
6-11 years........ 600 cals/d
>12 years......... 800 cals/d

- Dietary supplements if indicated need to be given 2-3 times a day after meals or at bed time.
- Care should be taken to avoid excessive supplementation as it can hamper the child's appetite.
- These should not be used as substitutes for meals, but as supplements only.
- High protein supplements indicated for adults should be used with caution as they may not always suit the pediatric patient.
- Supplements with milk shakes require enzymes along with.
- An idea of the possible high fat, high carbohydrate and high protein foods can be had from those listed in Table 7.4.

Electrolyte Supplementation

Children with CF are prone to salt depletion with excessive fluid and water losses, leading to hypokalemia, hypochloremia and metabolic acidosis. This problem is aggravated especially in hot tropical weather; therefore, it is essential that children should be encouraged to consume plenty of fluids spread over the day along with high salt foods. Significant hyponatremeia may be accompanied by vomiting. The doses of salt recommended arbitrarily are as given in Table 7.5.[16] Breastfed babies are prone to get hyponatrmeic due to its low sodium content, therefore in some centers, routine supplementation of salt is practiced. Urinary sodium should be checked if babies show poor weight gain.

Table 7.4: List of Food Options for Children with Cystic Fibrosis

High Fat Foods	*High Carbohydrate Foods*	*High Protein Foods*
Spreads high in PUFA/MUFA instead of low spreads (sunflower/olive/ricela), on bread/ toasts/potatoes/vegetables. Frying foods instead of baking, grilling, and boiling. Chocolates, crisps, cream cakes, biscuits, buns, cream added to porridge, drinks, cereals, soups, ice cream, trifle, pastries	Potatoes, bread, cereals, rice, noodles, pizza. Breakfast cereals/sandwiches, potatoes, pasta, rice added to salads, fried rice, potato wafers, savoury, biscuits/bread, cheese sandwiches, sweets after meals, sugar in beverages, milk drinks, cereal puddings, kheer, jam, honey, chocolate spreads on bread, roti, squashes, fruits juices, fizz drinks, fruit custard	Beans (rajma), baked or as curry, baked beans with butter toast, nuts, peanuts, dry fruits, fish, eggs, chicken, meat, milk (full cream), cheese sandwiches, grated cheese in vegetables, soups, scrambled eggs, extra cheese on pizza, burgers, cheese slices in between munchies, full cream yoghurt.

Table 7.5: Guidelines for sodium supplementation in children with cystic fibrosis*

0-1 year	2 mmols/Kg (Nacl soln)
1-5 years	1 × 600 mg (10 mmol Na tabs)
6-11 years	2 × 600 mg (20 mmol Na tabs)
>11 years	3 × 600 mg (30-40 mmol Na tabs)

*Refer. Gavin JE. Nutritional management. In: Pediatric Guidelines for CF Care[16]

Table 7.6: Food diary of a child with cystic fibrosis

Date: Weight: (Kg) Height: (cm)

Time	*Food Description/type of preparation*	*Amount taken (raw measure)*	*Enzyme (Creon)*
Early Morning			
Breakfast			
Tiffin			
Lunch			
Evening			
Dinner			
Bed Time			
Any other (in between snack/drink)			

One way to ensure that the child is being maintained on adequate nutritional intake as per the desired amounts is to ask the parents or care-givers to maintain a food diary of the child. This could include all foods/drinks/beverages consumed throughout the day, which could be recorded datewise with a brief description of the method of preparation or type of food, or source of the food item in terms of any standard household measures, e.g. teaspoons, glass, cups, etc. A record of the enzyme taken along with which meal and the dose can also be recorded (Table 7.6). This record can be maintained about 3-4 days before the scheduled follow-up visit with the doctor/dietician. A glance at this diary can help the dietician assess the actual intake of the child and any modification in the dosage of the enzyme or the diet can then be suitably advised.

Vitamin and Mineral Supplements

Although fat soluble vitamin deficiency may be expected in children with CF due to high fat losses in stools, clinical signs of vitamins A, D or K are not commonly seen. However, due to low levels of serum vitamin E levels encountered in such patients, supplementation of vitamin E is recommended (5-10 IU/Kg/d).

Trace Elements

Iron supplementation is known to interfere with pancreatic enzyme supplements; therefore, care should be taken not to administer iron supplements in close proximity to PES.[17]

Absorption of zinc is also known to be affected in patients with CF due to fat malabsorption, due to the formation of zinc forming complexes with fat and phosphorous. Supplementation 5-10 mg/d of zinc can improve absorption effectively.

Other trace elements like carnitine and taurine are also known to have a beneficial effect on the absorption of fat. Carnitine acts by prevention of toxic accumulation of long chain fatty acids in the cytoplasm and of acyl CoA in the mitochondria. Taurine has been shown to decrease fecal fatty acids and sterol excretion, and also known to decrease the severity of steatorrhea.

Route of Feeding

Enteral feeding or feeding via a nasogastric tube is practiced in many Centers in the UK to build up children with CF and even in teenagers reflecting deteriorating nutritional status. However, it is not so aggressively practiced among the Indian Centers where children are diagnosed as CF unless there is acute problem of oral feeding amongst them.

Enteral feeding has shown to improve body fat, height, lean body mass and muscle mass, increase total body, etc. The duration of tube feeding may continue for a period of 1 year to longer depending upon the nutritional status of the child in terms of their nutritional scores.

For children requiring long-term enteral feeding, mostly a percutaneous endoscopic gastrostomy (PEG) is done which makes it convenient for both the patient and the caregiver. In some situations, the child is allowed to have an ad lib diet during the daytime orally and the deficit is made up by giving high energy nocturnal feeds through the gastrostomy. The common practice followed by most CF Centers in the U.K. Is feeding for 8-10 hours overnight with 1-2 hours break before the physiotherapy session in the morning.

Pancreatic Enzyme Supplementation (PES)

Apart from dietary intervention, the second most crucial aspect of nutritional management of such patients is supplementing their diets with pancreatic enzyme in order to make up the deficit or absent secretion of this enzyme by the pancreas.

PES is available as tablets/capsules of the enzyme which are an extract of the pancreas and is meant to be ingested with meals. These are available in the form of powders or more recently and widely used as enteric coated microsphere enzyme preparations. The powder form was available as pancreatin powder and rarely used today. The main drawback of this powder was:

- Unpleasant taste.
- Can cause irritation to the infant's lips if got in touch with the skin as also to the mother's nipples while breastfeeding (the residual granules smeared on the baby's lips can irritate the nipples also while feeding.
- If mixed with formula milk or in a bottle, it may start digesting the milk and also clog the teat of the bottle.

The widely used enteric coated microspheric preparations are available as tablets known as 'creon', which has many advantages over the powdered form. The enteric coating protects the enzymes from inactivation by the acidic medium in the stomach, disintegrating to release the enzyme only when pH rises >5.5 in the duodenum. The enzyme so administered can achieve 90 percent fat absorption if given in correct dosage.

The microspheres can be mixed with a little expressed breast milk or formula milk and fed by a spoon or given on a wet finger. There may be some granules left lodged in the oral cavity of the baby, which can be dislodged by using a clean finger and rinsed down with a little milk given along with. The best and easiest way to administer these enzymes is to mix them with a small amount of fruit juice/puree (which will hold the enzyme in a gel form) and give it from a spoon at the beginning of a feed. The commonly used enteric coated microspheres are available in the dose of 10,000 IU of lipase per capsule.

Dosage of PES

The dosage of the enzyme to be given depends on factors like:

- Residual pancreatic enzyme.
- Enzyme supplements properties.
- Amount of fat and protein consumed.
- Pathophysiological factors.
- Stool output (frequency/color/consistency).
- Abdominal pain.
- Fecal fat studies.

Infants

The general acceptable dose for infants, when first diagnosed is approximately 400-800 IU lipase per gram of dietary fat or in other words ¼-1/3 of the capsule (10.000 IU) mixed with expressed breast milk (EBM) or in some fruit puree and given by spoon directly before the feed. The dose may be increase gradually depending upon the response to clinical symptoms in terms of stool output, absorption and growth. As weaning is initiated, the enzyme can be opened and mixed with any semisolid food and given before a meal. Parents are encouraged to begin weaning in the normal way by 5-6 months and all home based preparations can be made use of with liberal helpings of fat in them. As for normal children, it is advised that parents should encourage wider variety of foods in the diet of their children in order to get them accustomed to a healthy eating pattern well into their childhood and later.

Older Children

As the children grow, the enzyme dose too has to be mentioned keeping in view their increasing weight and fat intake. Initially 1-2 capsules of standard creon can be recommended with the 3 main meals, depending upon the severity of fat malabsorption. The doses can be titrated based on the response of individual child. Care should be taken to give an additional dose of ½-1 capsule with extra fat based food or supplement.[16] Overall, the dose requirements can vary from as low as 500 IU to as high as 2500 IU of lipase per Kg body weight. If stools are persistently greasy despite a recent increase in enzyme therapy, the use of antacids should be considered, e.g. omeparazole or ranitidine, which help to make the acidic medium more alkaline, thereby encouraging maximum enzyme activity at the appropriate site in the gut.[16] If the total dietary fat of the child can be assessed accurately, the dose can be fixed as 500 IU lipase of dietary fat. The recommendations made by the Consensus Committee on Cystic Fibrosis[17] have been laid down as given in Table 7.7, based on both fat intake and weight.

The maximum dose of enzyme should never exceed 10,000 IU lipase/Kg/meals, due to the risk of fibrosing colonopathy and constipation. Very high doses of lipase in the enzymes containing 22,000-25,000 units/capsule have been associated with the development of the above complication. Other adverse reactions noticed are severe acute and chronic reactions.

Administration of PES

PES should be administered with all meals and protein and fat containing snacks. It has been recommended that the enzyme should be spread throughout the meal to optimize mixing and minimizing partitioning of the pancreatic enzyme with the liquid phase of the meal, which empties more rapidly than the solid phase.[19]

Younger children should be encouraged to swallow the capsule as a whole at the earliest, usually by 5-6 years of age. But until then, the

Table 7.7: Recommended dosage of pancreatic enzyme supplements

Age group	*Dose*	*Adjusting dose*
Infants	2,000-4000 units lipase/120 ml formula or with each nursing Or 450-900 nits lipase/g of fat	Increase by 2000-5000 units lipase/feed as volume increases or if symptoms of malabsorption return
Children < 4 years	1,000-2,000 units lipase/Kg/ meal Or 500-4,000 units lipase/g of fat	Snacks: ½ meal dose; if dose appears above range, compare unit lipase/g fat.
Adults and children > 4 years	500-2,000 units lipase/Kg/ meal Or 500-4,000 units lipase/g fat.	Snacks: /2 meal dose. If dose appears above range, compare unit lipase/g fat.

Ref. 18: Consensus Committee, J Pediatr 1995;127(5):681-84.

only option is to open the capsule and add the granules into the feed. Care should be taken that the granules do not come in contact with the oral cavity of the child, inclining to chew them, thus causing ulcers in the mouth. Due to large variation in the amount of food consumed by younger children at every meal, it is a good idea to spread the enzyme throughout the day's meal. However, with certain foods like sugary drinks, fruits, juices or sweets, there is no need to add the enzyme.

General Guidelines for Use of PES

Keeping in view the specific mode of action of PES and its effect on patients, certain guidelines have been formulated which should be kept in mind when recommending them:[20,21]

1. Enzyme should be given with every meal, at the beginning and during the meal, rather than all before or after.
2. An extra fat based snack may require an additional dose of the enzyme, e.g. crisps, chocolate, milk shakes, etc.
3. Creon may be swallowed as a whole by older children but for younger ones, it can be opened and mixed with foods, jam, honey, juice or puree to form a gel.
4. It should never be chewed or crushed to mix it with the food.
5. It should be kept away from hot temperature or not left in a parked car outside in the sun to prevent the degradation.
6. The enzyme should not be mixed with very hot food or in food with pH of more than 5.5.
7. The expiry date mentioned on the packing should be strictly adhered to.

8. It is not required to be given with squashes, juices or cold drinks.
9. In case of excess gastric acid secretions, histamine receptor antagonists like cimetidine and ranitidine can help relieve the problem.

COMPLICATIONS OF CYSTIC FIBROSIS

Diabetes Mellitus

The most commonly associated complication of CF in children and adolescents is cystic fibrosis related diabetes mellitus (CFRDM). This occurs due to a gradual destruction of glucagons and insulin secreting cells in the pancreas. It is recommended that all children of 10-12 years should be screened for diabetes mellitus, especially when there is evidence of failure to thrive and at times of pulmonary exacerbations requiring IV antibiotics.[21] Management of children with CF having associated diabetes mellitus are managed quite unlike other children with Type I diabetes.

The recommended guidelines for management of such children are laid down as follows[20]

- Complex carbohydrates should be encouraged
- Normal sugar containing foods can be allowed
- Dietary fat content is not restricted
- Foods like biscuits, chocolates, crisps, etc. are allowed
- Sugar free drinks can be offered in between meals
- Regular meal and snack timings should be adhered to.

It is however important to maintain euglycemia which can be done by regulating insulin therapy rather than imposing dietary restrictions. The management should focus on consistent timings and carbohydrate content of meals and snacks, which can be achieved by three main meals and snacks in between. Carbohydrate counting is a good indicator to keep count of the intake. The total fat content of the diet can be up to 40 percent of the total calories. Monitoring of HbA1c (acylated hemoglobin) every three months is advisable. Early morning (1-3 am) glucose levels should be checked monthly (Dawn effect) to exclude nocturnal hypoglycemia.[20]

Coeliac Disease

Coeliac disease is one of the nonpancreatic causes of malabsorption which can contribute to poor growth. Dietary modification in such patients involves excretion of all gluten products from the diet (See chapter on Coeliac Disease).

ROLE OF FUNCTIONAL FOODS IN CYSTIC FIBROSIS

Fish Oil

Some recent studies at New South Wales, Australia have shown that fish oil supplementation in the diets of affected children with CF, alleviates many symptoms associated with the disease. It is believed that EPA (eicosapentaenoic acid) acts by modifying the role of leukotriene B4, which is believed to be the main culprit in the excessive inflammatory response to bacteria characterizing CF.[23] Some authors have also advocated the use of IV fish oil supplements in patients with CF. In a study at New York, it was demonstrated that there was improved lung function in children supplemented with IV fish oil emulsion, and no adverse reactions were observed in their subjects.[24]

Turmeric

The role of curcumin an active compound found in the spice turmeric has been recently been studied to observe its effects in correcting the defect in mice. The normal secretion depends upon the function of a protein called CFTR (cystic fibrosis transmembrane conductance regulator) and it is due to some mutation in the gene encoding that is responsible for cystic fibrosis. Curcumin is believed to play a role in correcting this defect at the cellular level and normalizing the secretory mechanism of various organs involved and stimulates CFTR chloride channel activity. It was shown to increase CFTR channel activity in excised inside out membrane patches by reducing channel closed time and prolonging the time channels remained open. Stimulation was found to be dose related, reversible and greater than 'genistein', another functional compound that stimulates CFTR. However, more studies are still required to confirm this hypothesis.[25]

REFERENCES

1. Fitzsimmons S. The changing epidemiology of cystic fibrosis, J Pediatr 1993;122:1-9.
2. Meenu Singh, Rajender Prasad, Lata Kumar. Cystic fibrosis in North Indian children. Ind J Ped 69, 2002.
3. Sokol RJ, accurse F, Abman SH, et al. Nutritional issues in cystic fibrosis In: Pediatric Gastroenterology and Nutrition In: ASPEN Seminars on Pediatric Disease Vol IV. Ballistresi WF, Vanderhof JA (Eds). London: Chapman and Hall Medical, 1990;273-95.
4. Goodin B. Nutrition issues in cystic fibrosis. In: Nutrition issues in Gastroenterology, Series # 27, ed Parrish CR. Practical Gastroenterology, 2005;76-93.

5. Berker LR, Russek-Cohen E, et al. Stature as a prognostic factor in survival. J Am Diet Assoc 2001; 101:438-42 clinical Practice guidelines for cystic fibrosis. Bethesda, MD; Cystic Fibrosis Foundation 1997.
6. Cystic Fibrosis Foundation. Clinical Practice Guidelines for cystic fibrosis. Bethesda, MD: Cystic Fibrosis Foundation 1997.
7. Metropolitan Life Insurance Company. Statistical Bulletin, 1983; 64:2-9.
8. Murphy JL, Wooten SA, Bond SA, Jackson AA. Energy content of stools in normal healthy controls and patients with CF. Arch Dis Childh 1991;66: 495-500.
9. Bell SC, Saunder MJ, Elborn JS, Shale DJ. Resting energy expenditure and oxygen cost of breathing in patients with cystic fibrosis. Thorax, 1996;5:126-31.
10. Slesinski MJ, Gloninger MF, Costantino JP, Orenstein DM. Lipid levels in adults with cystic fibrosis. J Am Diet Assoc 1994;94:402-8.
11. Peters SA, Rolls CJ. Vitamin therapy in cystic fibrosis- a review and rationale. J Clin Pharm Ther, 1993;18:33-8.
12. Leonard CH, Knox AJ. Pancreatic enzyme supplements and vitamins in cystic fibrosis. J Hum Nutr Diet, 1997;10:3-16.
13. MacDonald A. Nutritional management in cystic fibrosis: personal practice. Arch Dis Childh, 1996;74:81-7.
14. Green MR, Buchanan E, Weaver LT. Nutritional management with cystic fibrosis. Arch Dis Childh, 1995;72:452-6.
15. Anthony H, Smith A, Phelan P, Paxton S. Current approaches to the nutritional management of children with cystic fibrosis in Australia. J Pediatr Child Health, 1998;34:170-4.
16. Gavin JE. Nutritional management. In: Pediatric Guidelines for cystic fibrosis care. Hill CM (Ed); London: Churchill Livingstone; 1998;65-78.
17. Zempsky WT, Rosenstein BJ, Carrol JA, Oski FA. Effect of pancreatic enzyme supplements in iron absorption. Am J Dis Child 1989;143: 962-72.
18. Borwitz DS, Grand RJ, Durie PR. Use of pancreatic enzyme supplement for patients with cystic fibrosis in the context of fibrosing colonopathy. Consensus Committee. J Pediatr 1995;127(5):681-4.
19. Taylor CJ, Hillel PG, Ghosh S, et al. Gastric emptying and intestinal transit of pancreatic supplements in cystic fibrosis. Arch Dis Childh 1999;80:149-52.
20. Vavessa Shaw, Margaret D Lawson. Cystic fibrosis In: Clinical Pediatric Dietetics, Blackwell Publishers 2001.
21. Orenstein DM, Rosentein BJ, Stern RC: Gastrointestinal System and Pancreas. In: Cystic Fibrosis. Medical Care, Lippincott Williams and Wilkins, 2000, Philadelphia.
22. Beery HK, Kellog FW, Hunt MM, et al. Dietary supplement and nutrition in children with cystic fibrosis. Am J Dis Childh 1975;129:165-71.
23. Lawrence R, Sorell T. Eicosapentaenoic acid in CF: Evidence of a pathogenic role for leukotriene B4. The Lancet, Vol. 342, Aug 21, 1993;465-69.

24. Katz, David P, et al. The use of IV fish oil emulsion enriched with omega 3-fatty acids in patients with cystic fibrosis. Nutrition, vol. 12, No. 5, 1996;324-39.
25. Allan L Berger, Christoph O Randak, Lynda S Ostedgaard, et al. J Biol Chem 2005, Vol. 280, Issue 7, 5221-6.

Chapter 8 Diet in Constipation

Constipation in children is a very common disorder and is responsible for up to 25 percent of all pediatric gastroenterological consultations and up to 3 percent of all pediatric outpatient visits. It is estimate that in 90 percent of the cases, the problem is functional in origin while about 10 percent of them might have some latent organic cause.[1]

A systematic review of literature reveals a prevalence of constipation ranging from 7-29.6 percent both in Western and non Western countries.[2] According to Baker,[3] most of the time there does not seem to be any obvious anatomic, biochemical or physiologic abnormalities. A majority of them seem to be associated with functional factors resulting due to probable improper toilet training. Children usually have a tendency to with hold stool, either due to laziness, or preoccupation with playing or even after a painful experience of stool passage on earlier occasions.

Parents generally keep a keen track of the stooling pattern of their child, since this reflects his status of well-being, rather a healthy digestive system. This is particularly true for most mothers with children especially in their first 2 years of life.

The normal frequency of bowel movements varies with age. Infants pass a mean of 4 stools per day, which progressively decreases on an average, to 2 stools per day at 1 year and 1 stool every 2-3 days. But as long as the stools are soft and passage is painless, it cannot be termed as constipation. It may be defined as a delay or difficulty in defecation present for 2 or more weeks or as passing less than 3 stools per week.

Based on the type of presentation of symptoms,[4] etiology of constipation can be broadly divided into:

- Medical cause
- Surgical cause

IDIOPATHIC/FUNCTIONAL CONSTIPATION

This is perhaps the most common causes of constipation observed among children. The gastrointestinal tract undergoes changes in its physiological forms as the child grows from infancy to older age. The frequency of stool passage can be as frequent as one stool after every feed to almost 1-2 stools every 2-3 days in a breastfed child. As the child is introduced to complementary cereal based diet, the frequency and the consistency of the child also alters to 1-2 stools per day. To a large extent this may depend on how effective toilet training received by the child from the first year of his life. To term constipation as functional, certain criteria need to be fulfilled.[5] These are:

a. Two stools or less per week.
b. At least one episode of incontinence per week.
c. History of stool with holding behavior.
d. Abdominal pain.
e. Fecaloma in the rectum.
f. Presence of bulky stools tending to clog toilets.

MANAGEMENT

Children with such type of constipation require timely and prompt action on the part of the parents and the health caregivers. Proper toilet training at an age when the child is able to sit without support can help prevent such situations. A great deal of patience may be required to deal with toddlers as they tend to be restless and easily distractible. Training from an early age can help the child form a habit, so that by the time he reaches the school going stage, he is completely habituated to a set time to pass stool.

It is equally important to maintain a fixed routine for the child regarding his eating and sleeping pattern. Erratic timings of waking and sleeping also influence the gastrointestinal reflex to conform to a regular normal cycle of evacuation.

Stress is another factor which could cause functional constipation. It could be pressure on the child to get ready for school or in older children, the fear of an approaching examination or just disinterest in attending school.

The key to management lies in disciplining the child's routine in such a way that it does not impact the normal physiological functions like sleep hours, meal timings and bowel functions. Waking up late and consequently rising late can affect the eating pattern of the child thus disturbing the normal physiological cycle. An adequate diet with a good amount of fiber and residue can help maintain the normal bowel movements. Encouraging consumption of green leafy vegetables and liberal amounts of fruits, whole grain cereals and pulses from the early years will help them develop taste for these foods, and thus develop healthy eating habits. Excess consumption of milk and milk products, processed or tinned foods need to be curtailed in the schedule of the child's diet. Excess of milk in the diet also should be avoided as it can compensate for the solid cereal based food intake, thereby depriving adequate fiber in the diet. Apart from this cow's milk allergy has also been reported to present like features of Hirschsprung's disease.[4,5] Plenty of fluids in the form of water are equally important to maintain hydration, thus helping in maintaining the motility of the gut and softening of stools.

MEDICAL CAUSES OF CONSTIPATION

Apart from functional factors, occasionally certain other factors can affect the normal bowel movement of children. Among them hypothyroidism is a well known cause.

At times just electrolyte imbalance can also alter the normal functioning as in case of hypercalcemia. Dehydration is an important nonfunctional factor affecting bowel functioning.

Some other factors like medicines used for any other problems can cause constipation like anticholinergics, antispasmodics and certain resins (chlolestyramine).

Finally, dietary factors as already mentioned earlier have a definitive role in causing constipation. These may be summed up as:

- Malnutrition
- Anorexia
- Dehydration[6]
- Excess cow's milk intake
- Residue insufficiency (especially in older children)
- Celiac disease
- Cystic fibrosis (pancreatic enzyme related)
- Meconium ileus (at birth).

SURGICAL CAUSES OF CONSTIPATION

Certain infrequent causes of constipation could be:

- Hirschsprung's disease
- Colonic or ileal atresia
- Meconium ileus related to cystic fibrosis
- Chronic intestinal pseudo-obstruction syndrome
- Anorectal malformations
- Medullar and sacral malformations.

All of the above require surgical interventions where dietary support can help postsurgery

MANAGEMENT OF CONSTIPATION

Management of constipation in a child calls for prompt dietary intervention and education of the parents. The primary goal of dietary management is aimed at:

- Providing relief to the child
- Modifying diet as per the age and requirement of the child
- Education of the parents
- Behavioral therapy and lifestyle modifications.

Most of the problems of constipation among children are a chronic one thus requiring long-term management. Approximately 30 percent of the children even beyond puberty continue to struggle with symptoms of constipation like infrequent and partial stool evacuation and fecal incontinence.[7]

This can have a long-term debilitating affect on the overall growth and development of the patient, besides affecting his morale. It is therefore important to focus on the management in terms of diet and lifestyle to prevent significant morbidity.[8]

Treatment of chronic constipation involves 4 phases as recommended by NAPSGHAN (North American Society for Pediatric Gastroenterology, Hepatology and Nutrition.[1] These are:

1. Education
2. Dissipation
3. Prevention of reaccumulation of feces
4. Follow-up

Parents need to be educated, reassured and counseled regarding the normal stooling pattern of children which varies from that at birth or early infancy when the child is exclusively breast fed to older children when they are weaned off to a full 'family pot' diet.

They should be advised to refrain from blaming the child for his/her bowel habits. On the contrary, they should try to inculcate prompt toilet training, so that the child is accustomed in terms of his eating and sleeping habits.

Adequate and the right type of diet is no doubt one factor which can influence the bowel habits by a good proportion of dietary fiber, but it may not always be the sole cause for chronic constipation in certain children. Dietary fiber given in therapeutic doses may not always be acceptable by the child due to the high bulk form and difficulty in consuming it, besides not being very palatable. Therefore, it would be wise if parents do not insist or pressurize the child to consume fiber in this form. Rather the use of laxatives will help the child in passage of soft stools besides regulating the intestinal motility. Fears of side effects of prolonged or recurrent use of laxatives are unfounded since studies have not revealed any such evidence against them.[9]

Parents need to be reassured about the safety of such medicines used as laxatives in prescribed doses offered. The myth of osmotic laxatives having long-term side effects is in fact unfounded. However, a balanced diet with a good helping of whole cereals, pulses, green leafy vegetables and fruits still need to be complied with for long-term healthy gut motility, but of course without forceful implementation of fiber in the diet.[1]

Another factor commonly recommended is a liberal intake of fluids or water to improve bowel function with a view that increased amounts will help in smoother stool output. Actually, this again is another myth as indicated by various studies.[10,11] It is infact the solutes and not the water which contributes to ileal effluents; therefore minor increase in liquid intake will not help in altering stool consistency. Hence, it is recommended that unless there is evidence of dehydration, children with constipation should not be forced to drink more than normal amounts of water.

DISIMPACTION

This is done to remove large fecal mass present usually in children with constipation, to relieve the child of pain and discomfort. Rectal disimpaction is done with phosphate soda enemas, saline enemas or mineral oil enemas.

Recently use of PEG (polyurethane glycol) at the doses of 1-1.5 Kg/d has been found to be very effective and acceptable by both children and parents.

MAINTENANCE THERAPY

Use of laxatives to maintain soft stools and prevent constipation is usually recommended initially to prevent recurrence of impaction. Osmotic laxatives and PRG are used intermittently to prevent constipation.

BEHAVIORAL THERAPY

Along with maintenance therapy, behavioral therapy also is initiated for long-term results and maintaining regular bowel movements. Toilet training is encouraged by allowing the child to get on the toilet for 5-10 minutes daily if a fixed time after every meal. This stimulates the gastrocolic reflex allowing for an attempt to defecate. The child is asked to strain actively while placing his feet on the foot rest, thus avoiding holding back the urge to defecate. Children failing to respond to any of the combined above therapies are then referred to for psychological counseling.

FOLLOW-UP

Studies have shown that even after successful intervention in a child with constipation, relapse within the first 5 years was found in 50 percent of the treated children, while 30-50 percent of them persisted to have symptoms after 5 years of follow-up, even beyond age 18 years.[7]

To summarize successful management of children with constipation lies in:

- Education of parents and children about normal bowel habits and long-term adherence to treatment program.
- Use of PEG as first line drug in childhood constipation close and long-term follow-up in children with constipation to monitor relapse or persistence of symptoms.

REFERENCES

1. Constipation Guidelines Committee of the North American Society for Pediatric Gastroenterology, Hepatology and Nutrition: Evaluation and treatment of constipation in infants and children: Recommendations of the North American Society for Pediatric gastroenterology, Hepatology and Nutrition 2006;43:e1-e13.
2. Van den Berg MM, Benning MA, Di Lorenzo C, Epidemiology of childhood constipation: A systematic review. Am J Gastroenterol 2006;101-2401-9.
3. Baker SS, Liptak GS, Colletti RB, et al. A medical position statement of the North American Society for Pediatric Gastroenterology, Hepatology and Nutrition. J Pediatr Gastroenterol Nutr 1999;29:612-26.
4. Singh SJ, Arbuckle S, Little D, et al. Mortality due to constipation and short segment Hirschsprung's disease. Pediatr Surg Int 2004;20:289-91.
5. Kawai M, Kubota A, Ida S, et al. Cow's milk allergy presenting as Hirschprung's disease mimicking symptoms. Pediatr Surg Int 2005; 21:850-2.
6. Manz F, Weatz A. The importance of good hydration for prevention of chronic diseases. Nutr Rev 2005;63:S2-S5.

7. Van Ginkel R, Reitsma JB, Buller HA, et al. Childhood constipation: longitudinal follow-up beyond puberty. Gastroenterology 2003; 125:357-63.
8. Loening-Baucke V. Constipation in early childhood: Patient characteristics, treatment and long-term follow-up. Gut 1993;34:1400-4.
9. Muller-Lissner SA, Kamn MA, Scarpignato C, Wald A. Myths and misconceptions about chronic constipation. Am J Gastroenterol 2005; 100:232-42.
10. Schlessinger M, Fordtran JS (Eds). Gastroenterology, ed 6. Philadelphia, Saunders 1998;1451-71.
11. Debongnie JC, Phillips SF. Capacity of the human colon to absorb fluid. Gastroenterolgy 1978;74:698-703.

Chapter 9

Nutrition Support in Short Bowel Syndrome

Short bowel syndrome (SBS) is a complex condition which usually occurs following massive surgical resection of the small intestinal tract. The subsequent management of a child with SBS depends on a number of factors which determine the overall clinical course and nutritional outcome. These are the length of the remaining intestine, the site of resection, presence of colon and functional differences between small and large intestine.

ETIOLOGY

SBS generally presents in infants by birth due to a congenital anomaly or can also present later in older children consequent to any trauma. Intestinal atresia is the commonest cause occurring along the portion of the small intestine within an isolated area or along multiple segments. These can cause obstruction leading to GI ischemia, necrosis and resection.[1] Gastroschisis due to some abdominal wall defect can also lead to necrosis resulting in resection.[1,2]

In preterm infants, necrotizing enterocolitis leading to injury of the small intestine may also lead to SBS. Other factors like presence of pathogenic bacteria, aggressive feeding with hyperosmolar formulae may also lead to SBS.[3]

Malrotation of the GI leading to volvulus, is another cause of SBS in older infants and children resulting in occlusion of the mesenteric artery and ischemia.[1,2] Hernias and intussusception leading to intestinal hypoxic injury can necessitate resection leading to SBS.[1]

PATHOPHYSIOLOGY

In a condition of SBS, it is assumed that postsurgery, the patient is left with <200 cm of functional small intestine. The absorption is related to the amount of residual small intestine. It has been demonstrated that with as little as 15 cms of the jejunum and ileum with the presence of ileocecal valve, a good outcome can be expected clinically in terms of meeting the nutritional needs of the infant. However, without the valve, about 40 cms of the jejunum is minimally required.[4]

The site of resection of the intestine also determines the degree and extent of malabsorption. The duodenum and jejunum being the major sites for absorption of proteins, fats and certain minerals, cannot take on the functions of the ileum which is the only site for absorption of Vitamin B_{12} and bile salts. On the other hand, the ileum can adapt and compensate for jejunal loss. Therefore resection of the ileal portion can result in decreased enterohepatic circulation and malabsorption of vitamin B_{12} and bile salts and also the fat soluble vitamins due to impaired micelle formation.

There is malabsorption of the carbohydrates in condition of jejunal resection due to the loss of mucosa containing brush border hydrolases. Nonabsorbed sugar produce an osmotic diarrhea. The risk of small bowel overgrowth is increased, resulting in deconjugation of bile acids, mucosal inflammation and further compromising digestion and absorption. Reduced levels of cholecystokinin and secretion along with loss of jejunum contribute to impaired pancreatic and biliary secretion. There is evidence of N deficiency as a result of malabsorption and peptides and amino acids which further leads to impaired pancreatic exocrine secretion.

The proximal small bowel absorbs minerals like iron, calcium and magnesium and in the absence of this part of the bowel calcium and fat malabsorption combined leads to formation of insoluble soaps. This could result in increased absorption of dietary oxalates. Patients with colon in continuity with shortened bowel may be inclined to have hyperoxaluria and are at risk of forming renal oxalate stones.

In children with high stoma and fluid stools, there is excessive loss of micronutrients like magnesium, zinc, copper and selenium. Iron deficiency can result from loss of the duodenal jejunal area or from complications of ileocecal anastomosis.

Water soluble vitamin deficiencies like that of B_{12} and other B group vitamins occur in conditions of extensive loss of jejunum and ileum. Vitamin D absorption may also be affected in the event of loss of ileum. Unabsorbed fatty acids are converted to hydroxyl fatty acids by colonic bacteria and together with unabsorbed bile acids, induce colonic secretion exacerbating diarrhea.

Overall gut adaptation and functional prognosis is more of a challenge following ileal resection compared to jejuna resection. Ileal resection and the length of the remaining colon also can impact the course of the nutritional management and overall clinical outcome of SBS. Fluid and electrolyte losses are also increased due to rapid transit time. These can be better maintained if the colon is relatively preserved. Energy balance is also known to improve through colonic preservation as short chain fatty acids, a byproduct of bacterial carbohydrate fermentation in the colon, can provide up to an additional 500 calories per day.[5]

NUTRITIONAL MANAGEMENT IN SHORT BOWEL SYNDROME

Nutritional management is the most important aspect of medical management of SBS the goals of which being:

- Promote adaptation
- Maintain normal growth
- Avoid complications.

After resection of the small bowel, there follows a process of adaptation by the remaining intestine by the process of cell hyperplasia, leading to increased mucosal surface area. Besides, there is increase in bowel circumference length and bowel wall thickness, villous height, crypt depth, cell proliferation and role of cell migration up the villous.[6] For these adaptive processes to take place, good luminal nutrition is essential and should begin as early as possible.

The foremost consideration while managing a child with SBS is to maintain or provide adequate macro and micronutrients and fluid to prevent energy protein malnutrition and correction of acid base disturbances.

Ideally the nutritional management of a child with SBS is done in 3 stages although it may vary from one child to another depending upon a number of factors, clinical and physiological.[2,7]

The three stages are based on the requirements and physiological condition of the infants to be able to tolerate and assimilate the nutrients administered without any adverse affects. It begins with initially starting with parenteral nutrition (PN), which generally takes care of electrolyte and initial hydration. Gradually, the child is weaned on to enteral nutrition (EN), after initial stabilization and improved intestinal adaptation. In the final stage, which takes a time period of a few months to a year, the child is able to tolerate feeds and begins to accept orally well.

Stage 1: Parenteral Nutrition

In the case of pediatric SBS, central venous route is used to administer PN which can take care of the macronutrients requirements in the initial phase. Carbohydrates, proteins and amino acids are used in a balanced ratio suitable to the individual requirements to achieve optimal growth.

Parenteral lipids are infused at 1 g/Kg/d and gradually increased by 1 g/Kg/d. These should be maintained at around 30-40 percent of the total calories. This ratio helps to minimize the risk of hyperlipidemia, especially in small for date or stressed neonates.[6]

Carbohydrates are provided by infusion of dextrose at 5-7 mg glucose/kg/min and increased gradually by 1-3 mg glucose/Kg/min to a maximum of 12-14 mg glucose/Kg/min.[7] This way there is minimum risk of hyperglycemia due to gradual response of endogenous insulin. Excess carbohydrate provision can also lead to risk of excess carbon dioxide production and retention, besides preventing immune dysfunction.[6]

Amino acids are infused parenterally about 1.5-2 g/Kg/d and increased to the required goal gradually. Neonates generally tolerate amino acids well in progressive doses.

The requirement of electrolytes and minerals for a child with SBS is met by supplementing them with the PN. Pediatric multivitamin solutions are available which can be supplemented with the PN. Most children tend to have high ostomy output and diarrhea for which electrolytes and fluid need to be replaced in addition to the normal requirements.

Stage 2: Enteral Nutrition

Once the child is stable on PN therapy in terms of fluids and electrolytes, gradual initiation of EN should be encouraged. In new borns, EN is generally introduced as a lactose free based formula, preferably having protein hydrolysate. In the Western Market products like 'Pregestimil' from Mead and Johnson are tailor made and readily available. In the Indian setting in the absence of such formulae, there are a few commercially available formulae (like Protinex, containing protein hyrolysate containing 56.6 percent prtoein hydrolysate or Nova Source peptide containing proteins in peptide forms) which can be used as a protein source. Mostly the formula used in feeding, in infants and children with SBS are elemental, semielemental or peptide based, as in contrast to adult patients, where complex proteins are preferred due to their better promotion of intestinal adaptation. The reason is that infants and children are more prone to allergenic reactions if exposed to complex macro or micromolecules. Moreover, this can predispose to bacterial overgrowth and GI allergies.[8]

Initially the feeds are given as a continuous nasogastric form with a flow rate of 1 ml/hr, and slowly increased over weeks or months as PN is gradually reduced and tapered off. The advantage of giving continuous feedings is that the risk of emesis, abdomen distension and high ostomy output are greatly reduced. The rate of increasing the flow of EN would depend upon the nature and length of the residual bowel. The ideal mucosa is better able to absorb solutes against a concentration gradient than jejuna mucosa. Therefore in children with ileal resection there is increased likelihood of fluid and electrolyte losses. The earlier the EN is initiated, sooner is the likelihood of greater intestinal adaptation which refers to the process of cellular hyperplasia, villous hypertrophy, intestinal lengthening and enhanced hormonal response, thus facilitating greater absorptive surface area.[5] It has been shown that the process of intestinal adaptation can occur anywhere from 24-48 hours postresection, the entire process can take up to over a year to occur depending on the course of EN therapy and clinical response based on numerous physiological and metabolic factors.[1,2,9] With gradually increasing the strength of the EN, there is better intestinal adaptation, which can allow for further reduction in dependence on PN. But, in some infants, if there is evidence of increased diarrhea or ostomy output by about 50 percent, the increase in EN is usually contraindicated.

The preferred lipids are generally long chain fatty acids, since as compared to medium chain triglycerides (MCT), they have a greater potential for exerting trophic effect and promoting intestinal adaptation. Though MCT are more water soluble and hence have improved absorption, they have a higher osmotic load and lower trophic affect.[10,11]

Carbohydrates should comprise about 40 percent of the total calories since excess levels can exert significant osmotic effects, thereby exacerbating diarrheas. It has been recommended that if the colon is absent, the diet should include 40-50 percent of calories from complex carbohydrates, 20-30 percent of calories from protein and 30-40 percent from fats. If the colon is intact, the diet, the diet should be higher in complex carbohydrates and contain approximately 20-30 percent of calories as fat. The lower fat diet is useful for patients who have a colon, and especially for those who have had significant ileal resection, because malabsorbed fat causes steatorrhea and further fluid losses. In children with intact colon, higher carbohydrate diets are beneficial, as these can be converted into short chain fatty acids by colonic bacterial fermentation and utilized for energy. Lactose restriction is not necessary unless the patient is lactose intolerant.[12,13] Avoiding simple sugars is the most important part of dietary modification in SBS as these tend to increase the osmolar load to the GIT, resulting in secretory diarrhea. Therefore it may be summarized that in children with SBS, where EN is to be initiated, it would be prudent to use either a protein hydrolysate or occasionally if indicated amino acid based formula, with a high percentage of fat of the long chain triglyceride type (LCT) as the optimal enteral fed formula. However depending on the site and extent of resection and the remaining functional gut, some infants and children may also be managed very well with standard polymeric infant formula, as demonstrated by some workers.[14]

ROLE OF BREAST MILK

The role of breast milk in enteral formula has been considered due to evidence of increased GI tolerance and reduced duration of PN as compared to protein hydrolysate formula.[6,15] It was inferred that the advantage of breast milk could be due to its good source of immunolglobulins and growth factor, which could enhance intestinal adaptation.

ELECTROLYTES, VITAMINS AND MINERAL SUPPLEMENTATION

Infants require about 4-8 mEq/Kg/d of sodium to achieve normal growth,[1,7,8] and as per estimates there is usually excess sodium loss from high output ostomy or diarrhea. Therefore, supplementation of sodium in adequate doses is recommended. Liberal use of salt and salty foods has been recommended for patients with an end jejunostomy or ileostomy, as losses of sodium range from 90-140 m Eq/l.[13]

There are also excessive losses of fat soluble vitamins, A, D and E and minerals due to reduced absorptive surface area and steatorrhea, therefore pediatric multi vitamin preparations may also be considered for supplementation.[7] However, due to the porential toxicity of fat soluble vitamins, monitoring of serum levels would be advisable before supplementation. In children with ileal resection vitamin B_{12} injections are recommended on a monthly basis to maintain adequate levels.

ROLE OF FIBER AND GLUTAMINE

Fiber has been used with success in infants and children with an intact colon in the management of short bowel syndrome. The explanation given is that pectin and polysaccharides which are soluble fibers can help lengthen the transit time, thereby facilitating enhanced nutrient absorption, due to a longer contact time with the intestinal mucosa.[7]

Secondly, it is believed that short chain fatty acids which are produced as metabolites of undigested fiber, can induce a trophic effect on the colon and serve as a primary energy source for the colon cells. For patients without a colon, soluble fiber can be beneficial to thicken the ostomy effluent and prolong transit time.[14] Addition of 1-3 percent pectin to the semisolid elemental formula of preterm infants following bowel resection resulted in a reduction of reducing substances in stools and reduced fecal fat loss from 21 percent to 10 percent, besides resolving metabolic acidosis within 2 weeks.[16]

Glutamine, a nonessential amino acid in the body is considered to play an important role in enhancing intestinal adaptation in infants with intestinal immaturity or with short bowel syndrome.[7]

Stage 3: Introduction of Solid Foods

Oral semisolid foods may be initiated in children with SBS as early as possible coinciding with the recommended age for weaning in any normal child. To begin with, high osmotic foods or those with very high carbohydrates should be avoided. A high protein, low to moderate fat foods are generally recommended.[8] They are encouraged to take small frequent meals during the day and it should be chewed well. The deficit calories and other nutrients can be given as nocturnal EN in proportions as per their requirements. Children with an intact colon are known to develop oxalate and renal stones as oxalate are bound to calcium which restricts its absorption by the colon and is excreted in the urine, leading to stone formation.[2,14] High oxalate foods are colas, tea, chocolate, nuts, black tea, green leafy vegetables and strawberries. Fluids should be adequate enough to prevent dehydration.

The management of a child with SBS, may be summarized as follows:[17]

Stage 1: PN

- Stabilize fluid and electrolytes
- Initiate PN
- Increase gradually macronutrients to the desired goal.

Carbohydrates

- Dextrose starting at 5-7 mg/Kg/min.
- Increase by 1-3 mg/kg/min.
- Adjust calorie level as per requirement in older infants and children.

Protein

- Begin at 1-2 g/Kg/d
- Increase to goal by day 2 of PN.

Lipids

- Begin at 1 g/Kg/d
- Increase by 1g/Kg/d-3g/Kg/d (infants <2 years and
- 1.5-2.0 g/Kg/d (children>2 years).

Stage 2: EN

- Initiate continuous enteral feeds with appropriate by optimizing gut trophic stimulation
- Gradually wean PN
- Begin small intermittent feedings by mouth and proceed to nocturnal continuous feeding
- Begin appropriate electrolyte, vitamins and mineral supplement.

Stage 3: Semisolids

- Begin semisolids as for weaning by 5-6 months.
- Before introducing carbohydrates, stress on high protein, low to moderate fats.
- Supplementation of semielemental or polymeric formula orally with increase in take.
- Feeding evaluation by speech or occupational therapist.

NUTRITIONAL COMPLICATIONS IN SBS

Constipation could be one complication of SBS after cessation of diarrhea, especially in children with cerebral palsy. Excessive use of refined enteral feeds and inadequate fluid intake can also cause constipation.

Anemia can be another follow through in such patients due to excessive blood loss probably from the gastrostomy site, mechanical erosion from enteric catheters or associated stress ulcers.

There could be a risk of protein sensitive enteropathy, as due to anastomatic inflammation and bacterial overgrowth, absorption of intact proteins occurs across the gut. Secondary anemia could also result due to inadequate gut length for absorption of iron, folic acid, vitamin B_{12} and copper.

REFERENCES

1. Vanderhoff JA. Short bowel syndrome. In: Walker WA, Watkins JB (Eds). Nutrition in Pediatrics: Basic Science and Clinical Applications, B.C. Decker Inc Hamilton, 1997;609-18.
2. Jojnson MD. Management of short bowel syndrome- a review, Support Line, 2000;22(6):11-23.
3. Price PT. Necrotising enterocolitis, In: Grok-Wargo S, Thompson M, Hovasi Cox J (Eds). Nutritional Care of High Risk Newborns, Precept press, Chicago, IL, 2000;425-28.
4. Sibert JR. Small Intestine length in infants and children. Am J Dis Child, 1980;18:513-96.

5. Vandrehoff JA, Matyr SM. Enteral and Parenteral nutrition in patients with short bowel syndrome. Eur J Pediatr Surg, 1999;9:214-19.
6. Hughes CA. Intestinal adaptation. In: Tanna MS, Stocks RJ, (Eds). Neonatal Gastroenterology: Contemporary issues. London: Intercept 1984;69-91.
7. Serrano MS, Schmidt-Sommerfeld E. Nutritional support of infants with short bowel syndrome. Nutrition 2002;18(11-12):966-70.
8. Warner BW, Vanderhoff JA, Reyes JD. What's new in the management of short bowel syndrome in children. JACS, 2000;190(6):725-36.
9. Wessel JJ. Short Bowel Syndrome, IN: Groh-Wargo S, Thompson M, Howasi Cox J (Eds). Nutritional care of high risk new borns, Precept Press, Chicago, IL, 2000;469-87.
10. Vanderhoff JA, Grandjean CJ, Kaufman SS, et al. Effect of high percentage MCT diet on mucosal adaptation following massive bowel resection in rats. JPEN, (1984);8:685-9.
11. Vanderhofff JA, Blackwood DA, Mohammadpur H, Park JH. Effect of dietary menhaden oil on normal growth and development and on ameliorating mucosal injury in the rat. ACJN, 1991;54(2):346-50.
12. Matarese LE, O'Keef SJD, Kandil HM, et al. Short bowel syndrome. Clinical guidelines for nutritional management. Nutr Clin Pract 2005; 20(5):493-502.
13. Parrish CR. The Clinician's Guide to short bowel syndrome. Pract Gastroenterol 2005;XXIX(9):67-106.
14. Ksiazyk J, Piena M, Kierkus J, Lyszkowska M. Hydrolysed vs non hydrolysed protein diet in short bowel syndrome in children. J Pediatr Gastr Nutr 2002;35(5):615-8.
15. Andorsky DJ, Lund DP, Lillehei CW, et al. Nutritional and other post operative management of new borns of neonates with short bowel syndrome corelates with clinical outcomes. J Pediatr 2001;139(1): 27-33.
16. Hawkins R, et al. Pectin supplemented enteral feeding in the treatment of short bowel syndrome in two infants. J Am Diet Assoc 1995; 96(5):1010-22.
17. Sinden AA, Sutphen J. Nutritional management of Pediatric short bowel syndrome. Nutr Issues In: Gastroenterology, Series 12, pp 29-48.

Chapter 10 Dietary Management in Fever and Infections

Fever has been described as an elevation of body temperature above the normal, resulting from an imbalance between the heat produced in the body and that eliminated from the body. Fever, by itself is not a disease, but should be considered as a sign of any underlying infection or inflammation.

Fevers may vary in the form of manifestation like:

1. May be of short duration or acute, e.g. in colds, coughs or any upper respiratory tract infections or any other viral infections. Most of the infections whether of viral or bacterial etiology have one common feature that being fever.
2. May be chronic, or lasting for months and even may be of variable pattern, e.g. in tuberculosis, enteric, viral hepatitis, diphtheria etc.

PATHOGENESIS

Fever, be it as a result of any cause, involves certain metabolic affects, which are proportional to the elevation of the body temperature and the length of time the temperature persists. Some of the metabolic affects are:

1. An increase in the basal metabolic rate which is almost 7 percent for every degree rise in temperature.
2. Decreased glycogen stores from the adipose tissue.
3. Increased catabolism of proteins, e.g. in enteric fever, viral hepatitis which exert an increased renal load by increase in nitrogenous wastes.
4. Accelerated loss of body fluids owing to increased perspiration and excretion of wastes.
5. Increased excretion of sodium and potassium.
6. The gastrointestinal metabolism too is altered due to altered motility of the gastrointestinal tract. Vomiting, if accompanied by fever can cause further imbalance of electrolytes and fluids.

DIETARY MANAGEMENT

During the course of any fever, appetite is generally compromised, resulting in decreased intake. This leads to the child getting lethargic and weak. It is essential that adequate nutrients are provided during this period, as this will prevent him/her from slipping into a catabolic state. The older concept of starving a fever no longer holds good; on the contrary this will only accelerate the catabolic state of the child and delay convalescence.

Energy

Due to the increase in the basal metabolic rate, the energy requirements are proportionally increased – almost 50 percent, if the temperature is very high and prolonged. Conditions like tuberculosis, viral hepatitis, enteric fever, pyogenic meningitis, liver abscess or empyemas all require energy dense feeding to prevent further catabolism. Easy to digest cereals and pulses prepared with moderate amounts of fat and/or sugar, honey, etc. can help to enhance the energy content of the preparations offered.

Proteins

Normal to high protein diets are adequate to meet the requirements in conditions like the ones described above. Milk and milk products, whey proteins, egg, chicken and fish are some high class protein sources which can take care of the increased requirements.

Carbohydrates

Due to depletion of glycogen stores during fever, liberal intake of carbohydrates may be offered which will build up the required calories. Sweetened beverages, but not aerated ones can help build up the glycogen stores. Fruits and fruit juices help provide adequate reserves of glycogen.

Fats

The intake of fats may be modified such that the calorie requirements are adequately taken care of. Emulsified fats in the form of butter or cream may be better tolerated as compared to heavy fried foods which may cause nausea. Too much of fried foods like snacks, etc. are best avoided. Contrary to the common myth that in conditions of jaundice due to viral hepatitis, slight increase in fat sources will actually enhance the energy intake and help in maintain the body reserves.

Minerals

Adequate amounts of minerals like calcium and iron also can be provided through the foods offered. Milk and milk products are good sources of calcium while green vegetables cooked along with the preparations can take care of the iron levels. Jaggery may be substituted for sugar, as it is a very good source of iron. Nonvegetarians may be offered half boiled egg or poached egg with bread which can provide both calcium and iron. Fruits and fruit juices can help compensate for the sodium and potassium losses which are very commonly seen in prolonged fevers.

Vitamins

Requirements of vitamins, especially the water soluble ones like thiamine and riboflavin generally increase due to the long-term course of antibiotics used to treat the infective fevers. This group of vitamins is generally not absorbed during the course of antibiotics, therefore it would be worthwhile supplementing them if oral intake is inadequate. Deficiency of these could lead to signs like angular stomatitis, cheilosis, etc. Good servings of fruit juices can help prevent such deficiency states.

Fluids

Due to losses of fluid from the skin via perspiration, it is essential to provide liberal fluid intake in the form of milk, juices, soups, buttermilk and water. Tea is best avoided in the case of infants and children as it is likely to cause gastric acidity on an empty stomach, besides suppressing appetite. Adequate fluid intake also can help maintain adequate urine output which facilitates waste excretion.

FACTORS INVOLVED IN FEEDING

The type of food offered would be determined by the age of the child, the type of illness, and of course the child's individual preference also should be taken into consideration. Small frequent feeding can be tried in case the child seems disinclined to eat anything. Taboos like 'hot' or 'cold ' foods or 'light' or 'heavy' foods should be broken and anything the child desires may be offered; e.g. rice is considered cold and avoided during fever or gram flour is considered hot or heavy and so not given. In fact, 'besan sheera' is a good option for a child with fever, being a good protein and energy source. Similarly banana is considered to be causing phlegm and so avoided, whereas on the contrary it is one of the most safe and nutritious fruits which can be given in almost any condition. Citrus fruits which are a good source of ascorbic acid and good antioxidants are generally avoided due to the fear of causing throat infection or is considered cold. Such myths only further deteriorate the already cachectic state of the child and result in delayed convalescence.

The consistency of the food offered may be modified as per the child's individual acceptance and suitability. Very high fiber foods may be avoided to facilitate easy digestion.

DIETS IN SPECIFIC CONDITIONS

Fever may be prolonged in certain specific conditions as the ones mentioned below.

Tuberculosis

In this condition, fever may persist for quite sometime despite initiation of antitubercular drugs. There may be associated anorexia too due to the fever, but attempt should be made to offer foods high in proteins and energy to compensate for the enhanced basal metabolic rate which increases the demand upon the body. Inadequate feeding is likely to lead the child to not only inadequate weight gain but also to weight loss. Consequently the child becomes quite emaciated with decreased muscle mass leading to a state of lethargy, decreased immunity and loss of stamina to perform the routine chores.

A high energy, high protein diet is recommended for tissue building besides the normal growth and development. First class proteins like milk and eggs should be encouraged. Other protein rich sources like pulses, especially soyabean can also be incorporated in the meal planning. If required protein supplements may be considered. Fruits and juices also should be a part of the meal to provide the much needed antioxidants.

Enteric Fever

In the earlier times severe dietary restrictions were imposed in children with enteric fever (typhoid fever), with the view to give 'rest' to the intestines. But it was realized that such restrictions further deteriorated the condition causing prolonged delay in the healing process. All essential nutrients were deprived of resulting in completely emaciating the patient. Only foods like barley water, rice kanjee, weak tea, diluted milk, buttermilk or flavored water, etc. were fed for the entire period of illness. In case of children whose physiological demands are at the peak such restrictions only lead to delayed or stunted development and growth failure.

It is therefore recommended that a complete normal diet as per requirements for the age of the child needs to be encouraged. A full balanced diet with all the food groups incorporated in different preparations can be offered to bring variety to the diet. Most important the food preferences of the child should be the basis of meal planning in this condition. Any kind of food taboos or myths should be done away with.

Viral Hepatitis

Jaundice is commonly encountered among school going children which is mostly of viral etiology. Fever persists for a prolonged length of time and typically there is severe anorexia in most patients. Again due to certain food taboos many foods are avoided in this condition, especially fats. They are mostly made to thrive on boiled food and that too most of the yellow colored foods are avoided. Thus the food presented is a very bland looking and tasting equally bland, which only helps in creating more aversion to an already anorexic child. Here too the requirements are increased for the healing of the liver cells and restoring the liver to its normal function. Therefore, a calorie dense diet with normal to high proteins and equally high fat diet should be planned to be able to meet the increased demands. Foods like milk based (casein) sweets (khoya), cheese, paneer, chocolates and such other tempting stuff can be given liberally to meet the requirements with minimum quantity (See Chapter 15). As mentioned for earlier conditions, anything that the child demands as per his/her taste can be offered. No food restrictions should be imposed. The only caution to be taken is that the food procured should be from a hygienic source, especially fruit juices or other snacks. Fried foods also may be offered if the child so demands, but fats like butter or cream are better options as these can be incorporated in different foods planned.

Finally the concept of 'starving a fever' would only translate in 'starving the child'.

Chapter 11 Nutrition Support in Juvenile Diabetes Mellitus

The increasing incidence of type 1 diabetes among children in our country is posing a major challenge to the medical community. The changing lifestyle patterns in terms of urbanization or modernization has brought along with, its own risks. Several studies have already confirmed some association between incidence of type 1diabetes with many nutrients and accompanying food additives.[1,2]

Some authors have also shown evidence of corelation between incidence of type 1 diabetes and cow's milk intake by the child in early infancy.[3-6] Reports also have confirmed that exposure to cow's milk before 3 months of age and having the high risk genotype resulted in an 11 fold increased risk of Insulin dependent diabetes mellitus (IDDM) compared with subjects with no risk factors.[7] Eating pattern in childhood has also been associated with type 1 diabetes at the population level. It was also observed that average daily intake of energy from animal origin like dairy products and meat, directly corelated with energy from vegetable food items like cereals.[8] It has been reported that over nutrition early in life may lead to hyperinsulinism thus acting as a predisposing factor for type 1 diabetes.[9,10] Though there are studies to confirm a direct co relation between long duration of breastfeeding and decreased risk of IDDM,[11,12] certain authors have failed to collaborate the findings.[10] One of the first observational studies from Finland showed that the age of introduction of dairy products is associated with risk of IDDM independent of total duration of breastfeeding.[13] In other words the length of exclusive breastfeeding might have some protective role against risk of type 1 diabetes.

Children have characteristics and needs that dictate different standards of care. The management of diabetes in children involves considerations taking major differences between children of various ages and adults. For instance, insulin dose based only on body size are likely to be incorrect; the consequences of hypoglycemic events are distinctly different between adults and children; risks for diabetic complications are influenced by puberty and the targets of education need to be adjusted to the age and development stage of the patient with diabetes and must include the parents or the caregiver.

The parents of a child who is first diagnosed as having a chronic disease like diabetes (including the child) are initially shocked and devastated. They may even feel a sense of guilt and repent their actions of having allowed the child eat sweets excessively. Or some of them who have had a family history might feel guilty of having passed on 'the bad genes' to the child.

An effective family based dietary education program targeted at the dietary modification of the child and their eating habits can only begin when parents are allowed to grieve and come to terms with the diagnosis of their child. It is vital to develop a rapport with the family for an effective and consistent dietary management. Young children including the school aged ones are unable to provide their own diabetes care and middle school and high school students should not be expected to independently provide all of their own diabetes care. Therefore education regarding diabetes care must be provided to the entire family unit, emphasizing age and developmentally appropriate self-care and integrating this into the child's diabetes management.[14]

The aim should be a gradual transition toward independence in management through middle school and high school.

DIAGNOSIS/PRESENTATION

Although the diagnosis of type 1 diabetes mellitus is quite simple and straightforward, it may be missed out, since the parents may not recognize the symptoms to be of significant concern initially (polyurea, polyphagia, polydypsia and weight loss). Only when the child is perhaps brought for some other problem or for not gaining weight despite eating well, is the problem clinched after a routine screening test. Another accidental discovery of the disease in children is made when the child is brought to the Emergency for diabetic ketoacidosis (DKA), which may occur even in the absence of the above-mentioned symptoms.

The American Diabetic Association (ADA) has laid down the criteria for classifying and diagnosing type 1 diabetes in their Position Statement (2004) as given in Table 11.1.[15]

In the absence of unequivocal hyperglycemia these criteria should be confirmed by a repeat test on a different day. The oral glucose tolerance test is not recommended in routine use, but may be required in the evaluation of patients when diabetes is still suspected despite normal fasting glucose.

Table 11.1: Criteria for diagnosis of type 1 diabetes

1.	Symptoms of diabetes and a casual plasma glucose > 200 mg/dl. Casual is defined as any time of the day without regard to time since last meal. The classic symptoms of diabetes mellitus include-polyuria, polydipsia and enexplained weight loss OR
2.	Fasting plasma glucose ≥ 126 mg/dl. Fasting is defined as no caloric intake for at least 8 hours Or
3.	2-hr plasma glucose ≥200 mg/dl during an oral glucose tolerance test. The test should be performed as described by the WHO, using a glucose load of 75 g anhydrous glucose dissolved in water or 1.75 g/Kg body weight is ≤ 18 Kg.

Refer. ADA[15]

In case of symptomatic children, in whom screening is done as a routine, (FPG) 120 mg/dl or a 2-hour plasma glucose ≥ 200 mg/dl, the test should be repeated on the second day to confirm diagnosis. However, in a child symptomatic for diabetes, a random plasma glucose ≥200 mg/dl does 'not' require a repeat test.

Glucose tolerance test (GTT) is rarely required in children except when the symptoms are atypical or where plasma glucose values are normal and the diagnosis is uncertain. Type 1 symptoms may present as incidental glycosuria or in an extreme form as diabetic ketoacidosis (DKA). This condition is usually seen in slender prepubertal age group of children. Almost 30 percent of the type 1 diabetes is known to present with DKA.[16]

MEDICAL NUTRITION THERAPY (MNT) IN TYPE 1 DIABETES MELLITUS

The nutritional needs of children with type 1 diabetes do not differ from those of healthy children. Children with diabetes do not require special food, nor do they need different amounts of vitamins and minerals.[17]

The total caloric intake should be based on the daily requirements of all nutrients based on the individual age which are appropriate for their growth and development.

Type 1 diabetics have to match their food intake to the anticipated time of eating, as they are on injectable insulin. Therefore the timings of their meals and snack consumption should be at regulated intervals and should be consistent with respect to total number of calories and proportion of carbohydrates, proteins and fats in each meal. As these children are on insulin which is released continuously from the site of injection, care must be taken that the timings of their food and snack intake is spaced such that the child does not land into hypoglycemia between the 3 main meals. Therefore, where intermediate acting insulin is used, in between snacks and a snack at bed time is advocated to prevent hypoglycemia. Similarly, adjustments of their meal pattern should be considered with respect to the activity levels of the child, either planned or spontaneous or even in the event of unexpected illness. All these factors require a well chalked out comprehensive nutrition education and counseling program which forms an important aspect of any successful management of type 1 diabetes in children.

GOALS OF NUTRITION THERAPY

The main objectives of tackling a child with type 1 diabetes are:
- To maintain blood glucose levels as near as possible.
- To achieve an ideal weight for height and promote normal physical and emotional growth and development.
- To prevent or ameliorate the complications of diabetes which are responsible for most morbidities and mortalities in such patients.
- To inculcate good dietary habits for good health.

The first objective being that of maintaining normoglycemia to prevent long-term complications, a controlled diet intake has short-term benefits in avoiding large swings of blood glucose levels allows easier stabilization and minimizes episodes of hypoglycemia and ketoacidosis. This may seem a difficult task for the parents to follow as is for the child, all the same it has to be impressed upon them that a 'free diet' has its own problems in a way that it may become over restricted in carbohydrates especially where parents might curtail to an extent more than desired by eliminating many foods, or the opposite can happen resulting in excess intake. The need is for a regulated carbohydrate intake with increased dietary fiber in order to lengthen the postprandial glucose curves, thus avoiding hyperglycemic peaks and urinary loss. There is no evidence to suggest that a low carbohydrate intake is beneficial, but quite a bit to suggest that it is harmful.[18]

Energy Requirement

Mostly a child diagnosed with Type 1 diabetes for the first time presents with weight loss, therefore, the dietary prescription should begin with estimating calorie requirements to restore and maintain an appropriate body weight and allow for normal growth and development. Of course the calorie requirement will vary with age, height, weight and sex as well as physical activity, season of the year and stage of puberty. As per the American Dietetic Association (ADA) position Statement,[20] the nutrient recommendations for children and adolescents are based on requirements for all healthy children and adolescents as there is no research on this aspect so far. They should adopt a healthy life style which ensures adequate intake of all vitamins and minerals along with a good fiber and moderate fat content. According to a study on dietary intake of 4-9 years old children with type 1 diabetes, in 1996, it was found that although the calories, vitamins and minerals were adequate, the fiber intake was low.[20] Moreover, most of them consumed levels of saturated fats well above the National Cholesterol Education Program (NCEP) recommendations.[21]

Carbohydrate Requirements

The recommendations for carbohydrate allowances for children has been varying from 40-55 percent by different authors from time-to-time. Earlier 40 percent of the total energy was recommended from carbohydrates, but lately the British Diabetic Association in 1980,[22] and updated in 1992 (Dietary recommendations for People with Diabetes: An update for the 1990s[23] recommends at least 50 percent of the energy to be derived from carbohydrates mainly fiber rich polysaccharides. The British Diabetic Association has specific recommendations for children and adolescents with diabetes, according to WHO the total carbohydrates should never be below 40-45 percent of the total energy as is generally in a mixed family diet. The Committee on Nutrition of the ADA in 1986 has recommended that carbohydrates should comprise 50-60 percent of daily allowances of calories.[24] These recommendations are based on the fact that increase in dietary carbohydrates, without increasing the calories may actually increase sensitivity to insulin and lead to improved glucose tolerance in both type 1 and 2 diabetes.[25,26]

Studies using diets containing 60-85 percent of energy from carbohydrates have shown good control over the insulin dependent diabetes and well tolerated. With adequate treatment carbohydrate handling is resorted to a state similar to that of normal subjects.[26] In addition, distribution between carbohydrates, fats and proteins will differ depending upon the age of the child. Breastfed infants will obtain approximately 55 percent of energy from fats, 5 percent from proteins and 40 percent from carbohydrates, whereas, a 5-year-old may derive 35 percent energy from fat, 15 percent from proteins and 50 percent from carbohydrates. Traditionally, the concept of a diabetic diet was based more on a restrictive approach unlike in the present era, where a more holistic family based approach is recommended. Carbohydrates can be increased but from fiber based sources and proportionate reduction in fat sources is advised. Assuming that carbohydrates provide more than 40 percent of the energy, the formula used is –120 g carbohydrate +10 g for every year of life. For example, a 2-year-old boy should have 120 + 20 g (140 g) carbohydrate daily. His estimated average energy requirement is about 1200 calories; therefore a minimum of 47 percent energy needs to be derived from carbohydrates.[27]

CARBOHYDRATE DISTRIBUTION FOR JUVENILE DIABETICS

Most children of the preschool age group may find the bulk of the high fiber, high carbohydrate diet difficult to comply with, therefore to begin with a slightly lower carbohydrate with a little higher fat intake regime may be advised. Gradually, the high carbohydrate, high fiber foods can be introduced once the child gets accustomed to the diabetic regime. Adolescent boys needing almost 2600-3000 calories may even require 400 g of carbohydrates per day, which may be appropriate during the rapid growth period of adolescents. The same requirements may be lesser, i.e. about 200-300 g in case of adolescent girls who mature earlier and therefore may need lesser amounts.[28]

In short, if a child takes a regulated diet with selected protein sources of milk and pulses or lean meat/chicken, a moderate fat intake and a generous helping of vegetables and fruits along with prescribed cereal amounts, an adequate energy intake can be ensured, providing a good diabetic control with insulin.

Ideally the carbohydrate distribution should be such that it is distributed between 3 main meals and 2 mid meals and one bed time snack or drink. Bed time snack is a good idea and recommended as it can prevent the child from going into hypoglycemia at midnight or early morning. It is advisable that this late night or bed time snack be of unrefined carbohydrate with high fiber content and some protein, e.g. a whole wheat bread sandwich or toast with a glass of milk. A list of Indian foods with carbohydrate exchange of different food groups are given in Table 11.2 (ICMR values).[29]

The distribution of carbohydrates also depends upon the type of insulin, e.g. short-acting, long-acting, intermediate or a combination of both. Generally, children treated with one injection of intermediate or long acting insulin with or without short-acting one, require approximately an equal distribution of carbohydrate between different meal timings and activity.

Current recommendations are increasingly supporting the concept of Dose Adjustment for Normal Eating (DANE) which implies that total carbohydrate content of meals and snacks is more important in determining the postprandial glucose response and this in determining the premeal insulin dosage.[30] The concept of carbohydrate counting is being encouraged in many centers dealing with pediatric population. This allows the users greater flexibility in the timings of meals, the amount of food eaten at each meal and the selection of specific foods. The objective of using carbohydrate counting system is to coordinate the food intake (carbohydrates) by matching the peak activity of insulin with peak levels of glucose resulting from the digestion and absorption of food.[31] This allows counting of only carbohydrates of the food, thereby allowing precise adjustment of premeal short acting insulin using an insulin/carbohydrate ratio.

The insulin carbohydrate ratio is based on the assumption that carbohydrate intake is the main consideration in determining meal related insulin requirements, together with SMBG.[32]

Therefore, it is now recommended that it is better to derive an insulin regime that suits the individual child's eating schedule or life style. It should be rather tailored to the food intake and not vice versa. So to begin with the care provider has to determine the right dose for an 'average' day of the child's routine, implying that the child be allowed to eat a normal healthy diet, maintaining the eating timings daily and using the blood glucose parameters, the timing and dose of insulin injection can be adjusted.

In the case of children and adolescents consideration should be given for the child's appetite when calculating the calorie requirements and nutrition prescription. The adequacy can be evaluated by following the weight gain and growth patterns as per the standard growth charts, on a regular basis. With holding food or forcing the child to eat without appetite should be avoided. But care should be taken to adjust the energy intake such that in case the child is overweight, it may be reduced and increased if the child has had initial weight loss.

GLYCEMIC INDEX

Glycemic Index (GI) is an important term often related to foods or diets prescribed for diabetics. GI is defined as the area under the blood glucose response curve for a specific food, expressed as a percentage of the area after taking the same amount of carbohydrate as glucose.[33] In simple words, it implies to what extent the blood glucose can rise after eating a particular carbohydrate diet, and these responses can differ from one carbohydrate source to the other. Foods with a low GI cause less of a spike in past meal blood glucose than those with a high GI. So much so that the response of blood glucose to the same carbohydrate food can vary if prepared in two different ways or given in two different forms. For instance, a pureed apple can cause a greater increase in GI or blood glucose rise as compared to when an apple is eaten raw as such. Similarly rice flour or ground rice can induce a higher response as compared to rice eaten as such in boiled from. This is because the effect of food is altered by the dietary fiber which might be broken down, or certain enzyme inhibitors like lecithin, phytates, tannins, fats, proteins or the structure of the food itself. Moreover, the GI of the same food has been shown to have varied response if eaten in a mixed form in a meal or when eaten in isolation.[34] Fruits and milk may cause a lower GI response as compared to most starches, while sucrose will cause a glycemic response similar to that of bread, rice and potato. But all said and done about various glycemic responses to different foods, the consensus now according to the ADA is that whatever the glycemic index of any food is, it is the total amount of carbohydrate consumed which is important, irrespective of the source of those carbohydrates.[35] It is therefore important that the dietician when counseling the parents of the diabetic child evaluate each meal as a whole, since the fiber, fat and protein content as well as the method of food preparation, influences the glycemic response to the carbohydrate content of the whole meal.

In general, cereals like wheat and rice and root vegetables like potato, carrots, etc. Have a high glycemic index (65-75 percent). Fruits have an intermediate glycemic index of 45-55 percent while legumes and lentils such as dried beans, peas, green gram and Bengal gram have a low glycemic index of 30-40 percent.[36] The glycemic index of various Indian foods are presented in Table 11.2.

Fiber

The role of fiber in a healthy diet was under rated in the past century, but gradually since the past two decades or so, a great deal of focus is laid on its importance regarding the physiology of the gastrointestinal tract like digestion, absorption and metabolism of many nutrients. There are mainly 2 types of fiber present in vegetables and grains- the insoluble fiber which includes hemicelluloses, cellulose and lignin. But there are a number of foods like fruits, pulses, vegetables, etc. which have soluble fiber (i.e. water soluble) such as pectins, guar and storage polysaccharides. Ingestion of any carbohydrates with dietary fiber results in a decreased rise in blood glucose concentration as compared to a diet with little or negligible dietary fiber like in processed and refined foods.

Table 11.2: Glycemic index of common Indian foods

Food item	*GI index*	*Food item*	*GI index*
Cereal Products		**Miscellaneous**	
Bread	70	Peanuts	13
Millets	71	Potato chips	51
Rice (white)	72	Tomato soup	38
Wheat flour	70		
Vegetables		**Dairy Products**	
Beans	79	Milk	33
Potato	70	Ice cream	36
Sweet potato	48	Curd	36
Yam	51		
Beetroot	64		
Dried Legumes		**Fruits**	
Soyabeans	43	Apple	39
Rajma	29	Banana	69
Bengal gram	47	Orange	40
Green gram	48		
Black gram	48		
Sugar			
Glucose	100		
Fructose	20		
Maltose	105		
Sucrose	59		
Honey	87		

Source: Jenkins etal. 1981; Am J Clin Nutr, 34:362[33]
Raghuram etal. Diabetes Bull, 7:64; 1987[36]

The British Diabetic Association recommends a fiber intake of 2 g/100 kcals/d,[36] but since this amounts to a very high bulk for children, an intake of at least 1g/100 cals/d has been accepted. This amounts to around 20-30 g dietary fiber in the whole day's diet which can be achieved by encouraging the consumption of unrefined cereals, grains and legumes, fruits and vegetables. Soluble fibers also have a beneficial effect on blood lipids, reducing LDL and VLDL cholesterol, while maintaining HDL cholesterol, while maintaining HDL cholesterol. However, very large doses of fiber too may not be always helpful as it can hinder the absorption of certain minerals like calcium, iron and zinc due to the high levels of phytates in high fiber foods. It is postulated that the attenuated rise in blood glucose concentration when a soluble guar is added to the ingested carbohydrate is due to delayed rather than incomplete absorption of carbohydrates.[36] On the other hand, cereal fibers which are mainly insoluble have long-term effects on glucose tolerance. Therefore patients with IDDM consuming a high fiber diet of at least 20 g of crude fiber, show improved postprandial glycemia but no change in fasting glycemia. The fiber contents of various Indian foods are provided in Tables 11.3A and B.

Proteins

The protein intake of children with diabetes actually remains the same as for any normal child. Any excess protein consumed above the normal requirement, enters the carbon pool and ultimately is converted into glucose or fat. This is about 10-20 percent of the total daily energy intake which works out to be around 0.9-2.2 g/Kg body wt/day. The protein can be a mix of animal and plant source. But care should be taken not to stress only on animal protein due to the risk of high fat content also of such foods like whole milk, meat, pork, etc.

Fat

Fat is essential to some extent in the diet of children and adolescents due to their ongoing growth and development besides providing adequate vitamins and essential fatty acids. Patients with IDDM and even NIDDM have also shown an increased prevalence of macrovascular disease, the main clinical consequences of which are atherosclerosis of the coronary, cerebral and large arteries of the lower extremities. Since excess dietary fat which includes saturated fat, cholesterol and total cholesterol, is also linked to an increased lipid profile, which is a major determinant of atherosclerosis, care should be taken that the percentage of fat from total calories should not exceed 30 percent, less than 7 percent from saturated fat and cholesterol not to exceed 200 mg/d. These are the recommendations laid down by the National Cholesterol Education Program step II (NCEP Step II) guidelines.[32] This can be achieved by encouraging.

- Use of skimmed or semiskimmed milk and milk products
- Reduced consumption of fast finger foods like wafers, chips and other fried foods
- Use of baked, steamed or grilled food preparations
- Use of fish and poultry instead of red meat
- Reduced total visible fat used in meal preparation
- Avoidance of 'topping up' food dishes with cream butter, etc.

Sodium

Sodium is commonly used as common salt in all Indian foods besides being present in all bakery products and other processed foods. As high sodium foods are strongly linked to metabolic diseases like hypertension, it is prudent to maintain the levels in the day's diet to a moderate amount of 2.5-3 g/d, which is also recommended for any healthy child.

Table 11.3A: List of vegetables with their insoluble, soluble, and total fiber content

Fiber food source	*Insoluble fiber (g/100 gram)*	*Soluble fiber (g/100 gram)*	*Total dietary fiber (g/100 gram)*
Bitter gourd	13.5	3.1	16.6
Field beans	9.3	2.1	11.4
Broad beans	7.3	0.8	8.3
Beetroot	5.4	2.4	7.8
Cluster beans	6.1	0.6	6.7
Green plantain	5.8	0.2	6.0
Carrot	4.1	1.6	5.7
Onion	0.9	1.1	5.7
Fenugreek leaves	4.2	0.7	4.9
Lady fingers	3.0	1.3	4.3
Cauliflower	3.5	0.7	4.2
Spinach	3.5	0.6	4.1
Potato	2.6	0.6	3.2
French beans	3.0	0.1	3.1

Table 11.3B: List of fresh fruits, nuts and seeds with their insoluble, soluble, and total fiber content

Fiber source	*Insoluble fiber content (g/100 gram)*	*Soluble fiber content (g/100 gram)*	*Total fiber content (g/100 gram)*
Fruits			
Kiwi	2.61	0.80	3.39
Apple, with skin	2.00	0.70	2.70
Banana	1.80	0.60	2.40
Pear	1.10	1.30	2.40
Strawberry	1.70	0.60	2.30
Peach	1.20	0.80	2.00
Mango	1.06	0.74	1.80
Plum, fresh	0.70	0.80	1.50
Pineapple, fresh	1.10	0.10	1.20
Grapes	0.60	0.40	1.00
Pomegranate	0.49	0.11	0.60
Watermelon	0.30	0.20	0.50
Nuts, seeds			
Flax seed	10.15	12.18	22.33
Almonds	10.10	1.10	11.20
Sesame seed	5.89	1.90	7.79
Brazil nuts	4.10	1.30	5.40

Source: (Re/ 37) Farhath Khanum, et al. Plant foods for human nutrition 2000.

This implies not making the food bland or unpalatable by restricting sodium too much but by restricting processed foods available in the take away joints.

SUCROSE FOR DIABETIC CHILDREN

A normal child usually consumes about 20-30 percent of his total carbohydrates in the form of simple sugar, which is incorporated in his milk, beverages and some other sweetened products like biscuits, cakes, ice creams or any other sweet. For a child newly diagnosed with type I diabetes, to stop sugar completely and at the same time increase his complex carbohydrates in the form of high fiber cereals, vegetables etc., may be quite a trauma, as would be for the parents. Besides, it may not be possible for him to accept a higher bulk in his diet, with the result there may be quite a dilemma for the parents to convince the child to eat and the child may just refuse to accept food at all. This could further destabilize his insulin regime and consequently pose a challenge for the family and the care providers to achieve his glycemic control.

In the light of this problem, many authors have now recognized that some sugar taken as a mixed meal may be safe without having any adverse affects on the glycemic levels, provided the amount of sugar is adjusted or accounted for in the total day's ration of carbohydrates allowed.[35-37] As already mentioned earlier, ADA recommendations also emphasize the significance of the total carbohydrates consumed rather than the 'source' of carbohydrates.[15] Therefore the inclusion of a controlled amount of sugar in the diet of children with type I diabetes can have some benefits like:

- Child is able to accept the diet which will not be too different from the rest of his peers.
- Dietary compliance becomes more easy and practical.
- Brings in more variety, palatability and acceptance.
- Can avoid use of sugar substitutes.

Sweeteners

The role of sweeteners has become quite significant in the diet of most diabetics for whom 'sugar free' concept is just impossible or difficult to adhere to. This seems even more applicable in the case of children who may be consuming at least 20-50 percent of their carbohydrates from sugars alone. In order to overcome this problem and to be able to achieve optimum compliance to the dietary regime, sweeteners have been well accepted and proven to be totally safe for both diabetic and normal children.[41] The sweeteners are available in two forms-nutritive and nonnutritive. The nutritive sweeteners are fructose, sorbitol and xylitol. Fructose is as sweet as sugar and is present as a constituent of many fruits and vegetables and honey in the form of free monosaccharides. However, these may not be suitable for children due to its slightly adverse affects on serum lipids. Sorbitol is a sugar alcohol (polyol) half as sweet as sucrose but, its use has been debatable to substitute in place of sucrose. Xylitol is also as sweet as sucrose and widely distributed in fruits and vegetables, but due to its adverse affects on the GIT, its usefulness has been debated.

Among the nonnutritive sweeteners, saccharine, aspartame and acesulfame K are commonly available and recommended by Food and Drug Administration (FDA) in the USA. Saccharine is known to leave a slightly bitter taste after consuming it, while aspartame, the most commonly used and recommended to be safe with an acceptable daily intake (ADI) being 50 mg/Kg/d. As per the FDA guidelines the amount generally used ranges from 2-4 mg/Kg/d, even if used consistently which falls well below the ADI.[42] However, in routine use I would recommend against using any artificial sweeteners in case of children, especially in order to guard against any unforeseen repercussions of its prolonged use. Moreover, once a child is given to understand that these sweeteners are safe for him/her, there is a tendency of their getting dependent on them routinely. I would recommend to teach the child to get used to not taking sugar at all, or in case occasionally even if he/she might want to consume simple sugar in any form it should not make a significant difference as long as the total carbohydrates are adjusted as per the weight and age of the child.

INSULIN REGIME AND DIET PLAN

Prescription of a diet plan for a diabetic is based primarily on the type of insulin regime that is provided to any child. The commonly used regimes are:[27]

1. Single dose of isophane injection daily (no longer used).
2. Multiple injection therapy: This involves 3-5 injections per day before breakfast, lunch and evening meal and isophane insulin before bed and or before breakfast.
3. Twice a day injection (one before breakfast and one before dinner).

This is routinely used and comprises mixed soluble and insoluble and isophane insulin or mixed insulin analogue and isophane insulin.

Isophane and isophane mixed insulin: Meals are planned such that the carbohydrates are distributed at regular intervals to avoid hypo or hyperglycemia. For optimum postprandial blood sugars the injection is given at least 30 minutes before a meal. Generally a five meal pattern of 3 main meals and 2 in between snacks and perhaps one at bed time in recommended.

Analogue and isophane mixed insulin: With this regime the meal plan is same as above except that meals can be taken directly after injecting.

Insulin analog in Multiple injection therapy: In this regime also meals can be had directly after injecting. This has a short period of action and so more appreciated by children and parents as in between snacks are not required, especially in teenage girls trying to control their weight.

Multiple injection therapy: This regime offers the advantage of more flexibility in meal and snack timings and the short-acting insulin is given prior to eating.

EXERCISE AND HYPOGLYCEMIA

The role of exercise in long-term control of diabetes in children and adults is well recognized. It lowers the blood glucose levels by increasing the noninsulin dependent uptake of glucose by the cells and increasing the insulin sensitivity. In case when children are involved in strenuous outdoor activities or sports, the amount of insulin can be decreased accordingly or additional exchange of carbohydrate say, 10-20 g can be given in some form of complex carbohydrate before an event or in some cases may be given even after (Sec Table 11.5 for CHO exchanges). In events like hiking, swimming or a game of cricket, extracarbohydrate exchange can be given in the form of some unrefined cereal, e.g. Whole wheat bread sandwich or cereal with milk as this will help to release glucose into the blood stream gradually. It is important for the parents to be aware that they should watch out for signs of postexercise hypoglycemia which can occur even several hours after the exercise, possibly extending to midnight. It would be advisable in such cases to give an exchange or two of unrefined carbohydrate with some protein base at bed time to avoid any such eventuality. A list of noncarbohydrate foods that can be allowed are given in Table 11.4. Seasonal alterations in sports activities and type of sports in which children are involved may need frequent adjustments to allow the child to participate in school team and individual sports. For this initially frequent self-blood glucose monitoring (SBGM is required to determine the dose of insulin to be adjusted along with the amount and type of food to be given. If blood glucose levels are < 100 mg/dl during the period of exercise, 15 g of carbohydrate can be given as a readily absorbable sugar. This can be in the form of electrolyte

Table 11.4: Noncarbohydrate foods allowed

Protein Foods	Meats........... Lean meat, chicken, fish, egg (white) Cheese......... Processed or cottage cheese (in moderation)
Fruits	Lemon, gooseberries, guava, avocado, pear, water/musk melon
Vegetables	Cabbage, broccoli, cauliflower, all green leafy vegetables, Radish, onions, mushrooms, beans, peas, tomato, salads
Beverages	Clear soups, lemonade, unsweetened tomato juice, sugar free fizzy drinks.
Fats	Fried foods and cream to be used in moderation Low fat spreads, vegetable oils, butter, ghee Grilling, baking steaming or pressure cooking to be preferred

containing sports drink. These are quite helpful in preventing hypoglycemia both during and after weight exercise. The dose of insulin may be decreased rather than increasing calories as this regime can help optimum weight management for all diabetic children. Studies in pediatric population have shown that discouraging sedentary activities such as television or computer monitors are an effective method to ensure physical activity and encourage weight loss in inactive children.

To sum up the recommendations for all children with type I diabetes are:[15]

- Children with type I diabetes should adhere to a minimum of 30-60 minutes of moderate physical activity
- SBGM before exercise should be done (parents can help in case of younger children). A suggested intake of 10-15 g of carbohydrate depending upon the age of the child can be given if blood glucose falls < 100 mg/dl; for vigorous activity of more than 30 minutes, additional 15 g of carbohydrate may be given.
- For prolonged vigorous exercise hourly blood glucose monitoring during the exercise as well as after the event is advisable.
- At the onset of a new sports season, frequent blood sugar monitoring during the 12 hour postexercise period should be done to adjust insulin dosage.
- Physical exercise (especially for overweight or obese) children and adolescents should be encouraged and sedentary activity discouraged.

Hypoglycemia is an important complication in most diabetic children and a cause of great concern to parents. It is generally a result of a temporary rise in insulin in the blood due to either excess dose or delayed or refusal of food intake, increased exercise or unusual exposure to cold. Delayed meals due to unscheduled assignments or emergencies can also contribute to hypoglycemia in which case it is a good idea for such children to carry a pack of some snack to be consumed to tide over such temporary crisis. The parents and children need to be explained common features of hypoglycemia to be able to tackle the situation promptly without landing into emergency situations as is commonly seen. These include sweating, pallor, and dizziness, restlessness at night or waking and altered behavior, e.g. sudden tantrums or depression.

Treatment of hypoglycemia generally involves giving an easily absorbable carbohydrate in a concentrated form, e.g. sugar or glucose. Diabetics are generally advised to keep some sugar cubes handy with them always. The dictum should be 'if in doubt, treat as hypoglycemia', especially so for a lay person who may not be sure of the hypoglycemia status. In severe cases, injectables like glucagon is required to be administered.[41] Glucagon reverses the action of insulin and is a secretion of the alpha cells of the pancreas. It is injected just like insulin and parents can be taught how and when to use it. It liberates glucose from liver glycogen, resulting in a rise in blood sugar thus reversing the affect of hypoglycemia.

However, parents need to be aware that children and adolescents may even take advantage of the existence of a state of hypoglycemia, which warrants immediate feeding. They may attempt to 'fake' hypoglycemia as an attention seeking behavior and getting sweets or any food of their own choice. In such situations a spot blood glucose monitoring can give a true picture.

CONSIDERATIONS IN DIFFERENT STAGES OF CHILDHOOD

Infants

Diabetes during infancy is generally of transient type and very rare. Insulin may be required in minimum doses. These children should have their carbohydrate allowances based on milk feeds which should be frequent and regular. Breastfeeding should be encouraged to be continued. Their fluid requirement of 150-20 ml/Kg body weight can be met by breastfeeds or top feeds (150 ml breast milk will contain approximately 10 g of carbohydrate). After 5-6 months complementary feeding should be initiated with noncarbohydrate sources like pureed vegetables and fed by spoon. As the child gets acclimatized to spoon feeding, carbohydrate exchanges from cereals and pulses can be initiated. To begin with, 5 g of carbohydrate exchange can be offered, e.g. 5 g of rice or 25 g of potato. By 10-12 months, the amounts can be gradually increased to meet the energy and protein requirements during their growth and development. By one year the child should be having about 90 g of carbohydrate as solids, the remaining coming from milk. Since the first year of life is the period of most rapid growth with constantly changing eating patterns, the parents need to be inconstant follow-up with their dieticians for periodic counseling and reassurance regarding the child's feeding schedule. They need to be counseled regarding signs of hypo or hyperglycemia. In conditions of recurrent hypoglycemic spells, it may be necessary to give cereal based carbohydrates (e.g. rice) earlier than 3-4 months to prevent nocturnal hypoglycemia.

Toddlers

Till 1 year of age whole milk can be offered but by 2 years semiskimmed milk can be started as by now the child would be on a full solid diet besides milk. This can continue till about 5 years after which skimmed milk or toned milk should be started, so as to reduce the total fat content of the diet. Gradually fiber rich carbohydrates can also be increased. There can be toddler food refusal syndromes and parents can face a tough time coping with their tantrums. In such cases slight variations in the menu or food choices can be made to avoid hypoglycemia. Too much fuss and forced feeding should be discouraged. After a long gap of food refusal with the child going into hypoglycemic levels, most often they accept food gradually. Most children on insulin feel excessively hungry- this could be due to poor control or sugar being lost in the urine. Re-evaluation of the dietary regime should be done and if required, adjust the dose of insulin as following the DANE concept.

School Children

By the time the child stares going to school, he or she should be taught to follow a prescribed diet schedule and become as independent as possible. The carbohydrate portions can be divided into 5 meals and snacks beginning with Breakfast, a mid meal packed snack and or a fruit till the child is back home for lunch.

The school teachers/authorities should be informed about the diabetic status of the child and be apprised of the importance of in between snack for such children to avoid risk and symptoms of hypoglycemia. If possible school should be able to provide suitable food or snack to deal with any crisis of hypoglycemia if at all it occurs. The child on his part also should be made aware of the importance of maintaining a regulated eating schedule and regarding the foods that he/she can take freely or need to avoid.

In case of social eating, the diabetic child should not be discouraged to participate, e.g. a trip going for a picnic or some children's party. However, school authorities or the hostess if at home, should take care to include some such food/dish like a sandwich, or some peanut packing, e.g. on toast or cheese preparation which the child can take. If parents can coordinate with the host regarding the menu offered, the child may be allowed to eat moderate helping from the party, and the carbohydrate counting can be adjusted in the latter part of the day, thus maintaining the recommended regime. Regarding consumption of sweets, children with diabetes mellitus need to be positively reinforced an explained the risks of going into hypoglycemia. They can be reassured that during exercise or some sports activity, some sweet may be offered. But still if the child is unable to cooperate or is on habitual bingeing, the services of a child psychologist need to be sought as this could suggest underlying stress.

Adolescents

Adolescent period being one of stress, exploring and rebellion, it might be quite a challenge for parents to cope with them and bring them to be convinced regarding their recommended dietary lifestyle. Snacking and eating out include use of alcohol and substance can be an added problem which needs to be tackled very patiently, yet firmly by parents and if required seek help of their psychologist or psychiatrist.

It is recommended that these children be appropriately counseled regarding the carbohydrate content of various portion sizes of various foods so that they can be aware of the choice of foods and also the importance of good control on their weight, e.g. a packet of chips may provide 10 g of carbohydrate and 150 calories, but an apple also will provide 10 g carbohydrates but only 50 calories. The carbohydrate exchange of various food groups with their portion sizes are presented in Table 11.5 (ICMR refer). This table can help the parents select and interchange equivalent foods within the prescribed amounts of carbohydrates and calories.

The prescribed amount of calories for children with diabetes generally ranges from 1000 kcals to 2000 Kcals or even more depending on their weight, blood sugar levels and age. Annexure 1 gives in detail the exchanges and their portion sizes along with calories allowed at different levels and sample menus recommended.

COMPLICATIONS OF DIABETES MELLITUS

The common complications occurring among diabetic children are:

Hypoglycemia

Main causes of hypoglycemia and its management are already discussed earlier in this chapter.

Table 11.5: Portion size of carbohydrate and calorie exchange of various foods

Food group	*Foods*	*Carbohydrate Exchange (g)*	*Calories (Kcals)*	*Amount Raw (g)*	*Number/Size*
Cereals	Rice, milled	20	100	30	1 serving (med)
	Rice flakes	20	100	30	1 serving
	Wheat atta	20	100	30	1 roti (medium)
	Wheat maida	22	104	30	1 roti (medium)
	Bread brown	15	100	30	2 No.
	Bread white	15	75	30	2 No.
	Suji	20	85	25	1 serving (med.)
	Dalia	20	100	30	1 serving (med)
	Maize, dry	20	100	30	1 Roti
Pulses	Beng. gram	15	100	30	1 katori (med.)
	Rajma	18	100	30	1 Katori (med.)
	Moong dal/whole	18	100	30	1 Katori (med.)
	Soyabean	10	200	50	2 Katori (small)
	Red gram dal	17	100	30	1 Katori (med.)
	Lentil	18	100	30	1 Katori

Contd.

Milk, milk products	Buffalo's Milk	10	230	200 ml	1 glass (med.)
	Cow's milk	10	134	200 ml	1 glass (med.)
	Curd, cow's milk	6	120	200 ml	1 glass (med.)
Milk, milk products	Khoa, cow's milk	6	100	25 g	1 cube small
	Khoa, Buff. milk	5	100	25 g	1 cube small
	Skim milk powder, cow's milk	12	90	25 g	5 tsp.
Roots and tubers	Potato	22	100	100 g	2 medium
	Onion, big	10	50	100 g	2 medium
	Onion, small	10	60	100 g	4 medium
	Carrot	20	100	200 g	4 medium
	Radish, white	6	30	200 g	1 big
	Radish, pink	15	65	200 g	1 big
	Turnip	6	30	100 g	2-3 medium
	Colocasia	20	100	100 g	4-5 medium
	Yam, ordinary	25	100	100 g	5-6 medium
	Arrowroot flour	25	80	25 g	1 serving
	Sweet potato	30	100	100 g	2 medium

Contd.

Vegetables	Brinjal, gourd veg/ leafy veg/ pumpkin/cauliflower/tinda	Negligible	Negligible	150 g	1 serving medium
Other vegetables	Beans, peas, tomato	10 g	50	50-100 g	1 small serving
Fruits	Apple	10 g	50	75 g	1 small
	Banana	10	50	30 g	¼ small
	Grapes	10	50	100 g	20 No.
	Guava	10	50	100 g	1 medium
	Papaya	10	50	120 g	2 slices, med.
	Mango	10	50	75 g	1 small
	Pear	10	50	100 g	1 medium
	Watermelon	10	50	175 g	¼ small
	Pineapple	10	50	100 g	2 slices round
	Orange	10	50	100 g	1 big
	Melon, musk	10	50	300 g	6-7 slices
	Plum	10	50	120 g	4 medium
Animal Foods	Egg/chicken/meat/fish	Nil	100	-----	2/75 g/75 g/75 g

Source: TC Raghuram, Swaran Pasricha, Sharma RD. Diet and Diabetes; National Institute of Nutrition, ICMR, Hydreabad 1998[35]

Contd.

Diabetic Ketoacidosis (DKA)

This occurs as a consequence of absolute or relative insulin deficiency resulting in hyperglycemia and an accumulation of ketone bodies in the blood with subsequent metabolic acidosis. It is one of the commonest causes of emergency admissions in a Pediatric Center. Quite often DKA is the first presentation of a child being newly diagnosed with type I diabetes mellitus. In a known diabetic child, the most common cause is omission of insulin dose, intercurrent illness, trauma, surgery or any other stress related factor. Children coming with recurrent episodes of DKA need special attention. These are the group who periodically default on their regular insulin injections or fail to adhere to the recommended dietary regime. The cause for this could be underlying eating disorders or depression which might warrant psychiatric intervention.

Illness and Hyperglycemia

Illness of any kind in a child with type I diabetes also tends to lead to hypoglycemia and consequently DKA. Vomiting, nausea and pain abdomen may frequently be associated in most children. In such cases insulin should be continued with the dose being either increased or supplemented with short-acting one. Dietary carbohydrates need to be continued or replaced with fluids of equal carbohydrate content, e.g. lemonade with sugar, milk, drinking chocolate with sugar or a biscuit or some soup with toasted bread and butter. These can be given orally in sips gradually over an hour or two and when settled, may slowly be brought back to the original schedule. If the child does not improve or vomiting persists, hospitalization should be sought.

During episodes of acute illness children avoid eating for prolonged periods. In such situations, blood levels tend to be high; therefore insulin doses should be continued. Carbohydrate should not be restricted to control hyperglycemia, but the insulin doses should be adjusted to the blood sugars. At least 70-80 percent of the normal requirement should be given. This can be done by small frequent doses of rapidly absorbed carbohydrates in liquid form. Cold drinks without fizz can be given to prevent dehydration. For instance, on a diet requirement of 180 g carbohydrates, which is otherwise distributed between 3 main meals and 3 snacks. 35-45 g carbohydrates can be given as hourly drink between breakfast and lunch, 45-50 g between lunch and evening meal and 50-55 g between evening meal and night time. A list of noncarbohydrate sources of carbohydrate food which can be given freely are listed in Table 11.4.

Hypertension

In adults hypertension is generally associated with diabetes mellitus and may not be commonly seen among children. Nevertheless, it is advisable that blood pressure monitoring be done for them too and any sign or symptom if observed may be managed accordingly as per the guidelines of DASH (Dietary Approaches To Stop Hypertenion) diet.[34]

SOMOGYI AND DAWN EFFECT

Somogyi effect is described as a rebound hyperglycemia name after the physician who first discovered it. The rebound is in response to undetected hypoglycemia (blood glucose <70 g/dl) which generally around or postmidnight. In response to the hypoglycemia, the body releases hormones, glycogen and epinephrine which send signals to the liver to release glucose stores. Consequently, the glucose level can swing too high to cause hyperglycemia. This hyperglycemia generally is detectable towards early morning. Now on monitoring the fasting glucose, a picture of very high sugars is perceived due to which the caregiver is prompted to increase the bed time or predinner insulin dose. This would further lead to midnight hypoglycemia and the situation can worsen leading to DKA. This actually was the result of too much insulin circulating in the blood. To ascertain whether, it is actually hyperglycemia, or just a rebound effect, the best way to test is to set an alarm for around 2-3 a.m. at night and monitor the blood glucose. Low levels of glucose at this point will signify the Somogyi effect. If this is so, it would mean, reducing the night time insulin and or, ensure a bed time snack preferably protein based; for instance, some cereal milk mix, cottage cheese or some nuts or even curd.

Dawn effect also has features of early morning hyperglycemia as the name suggests, but this is not due to rebound effect of hyperglycemia. Actually, this phenomenon occurs with normal subjects too when counter regulatory hormones like growth hormones, cortisol and catecholamines cause the glucose levels to rise. But, in diabetes, due to lack of sufficient insulin in the bloodstream, the glucose levels are not controlled, thus presenting with hyperglycemia in the morning. To prevent this phenomenon, it is recommended that a diabetic child:

- Should exercise or indulge in some sport later in the day, so that more of glucose lowering effect occurs at night.
- Limit bed time carbohydrates and increase protein/fat based snack (nuts, eggs, cheese).

Nutrition Counseling and Follow-Up

Counseling is an important aspect of management in children with diabetes. A positive approach to meal planning is to encourage family members and other support persons to follow the same life style recommendations as the child with diabetes. A close interaction of the parents or caregiver, the child and the diabetes team (which comprises the dietician, the diabetes educator/nurse) is essential to achieve the goals of management in children with diabetes mellitus. The significance of a diabetic team has been emphasized by the landmark Diabetes Control and Complications Trial (DCCT).[43]

The focus of counseling should be based on the goal of:

- Promoting positive behavioral changes.
- Provide healthy meals and snacks.
- Focus on healthy eating habits of the entire family.

The child should be included in the counseling sessions and be reassured that he/she will not be put on a strict 'diet' and may also have some of their favourite foods. They need to be impressed upon, that they are being advised simply to establish a healthy eating plan which is not just for him/her but for the entire family.

Parents can be asked to maintain a food diary which can include all foods and snacks eaten by the child. Initially the child may feel very hungry due to glycosuria, therefore it is important to respond to their stimulated appetite. The appetite of most children stabilizes by 3-4 days of insulin therapy. The concept of exchange list of various carbohydrate foods and carbohydrate counting needs to be explained to the parents/caregiver, to help them include a wider variety and liberty in choice of foods while meal planning.

The parents can be given general guidelines like consistency with timing, amount and types of foods and the relationship between food, insulin and exercise and their effect on blood glucose.

The following points need to be considered while counseling parents of a diabetic child and the child:[44]

- Parents should not promote distorted eating to maintain blood glucose control.
- Changes in food choices should be done gradually.
- Children should be include in the counseling sessions on follow-up visits, and be involved in meal planning.
- The child should not be referred to as 'diabetic'.
- Reassure children that many of the usual foods can be included in the meal plan.

- Stress healthy eating habits for the entire family rather than focusing on the child.
- Avoid negative words like 'cannot', 'do not', 'never', 'should not', because these can promote negative attitude and indicate deprivation.
- Omitting or including certain foods on the basis of one single high blood glucose reading is not advisable. It could be stress induced and in such conditions with reduction in stress, hypoglycemia may occur if food is omitted.

Continued nutrition follow-up and education are required every 6 months to 1 year as the child grows and develops. Over a period of time the family also gets trained and experienced in the nutritional management of the child, and the child too gets confident of managing his blood sugars based on his activities and eating pattern.

ANNEXURE 1

1000 Calories Diabetic Diet

Exchange Distribution per day

Food group	*Exchange*	*Amount (g)*	*Breakfast*	*Mid morning*	*Lunch*	*Evening*	*Dinner*	*Bed time*
Cereals	5	150	1	1	1	0.5	1	0.5
Pulses*	1	25	-	-	1	-	-	-
Milk/ Curd Toned**	4	400	1.5	-		1.5		1
Fruits	1	100	-	-	-	-	-	-
Veg A and B	2.5	250	-	0.5	1	-	1	-
Fats/Oil	2	10		0.5	1	0.5	1	-

*Pulse exchange is assumed as 25 g/portion size.
**Milk exchange is assumed as 100 ml/portion

Percentage Distribution of Calories

Carbohydrates .... 60 percent (148 g approx)
Proteins .... 17 percent (38 g approx)
Fats.. 23 percent (29 g approx)

Sample Menu

Breakfast

Milk/Curd....................................... 150 ml
Roti/Cereal .... 1/30 g

Mid morning

Roti/Parantha.................................. 1/1 small (no oil)
Vegetables .... 1/2 serving (Group A)

Lunch

Roti/Rice .... 1/30 g
Curd.. 100
Vegetables .... 1 serving
Fruit*.. 1

Evening

Milk... 150 ml
Biscuits... 2

*Fruit may be had any other convenient time also

Dinner

Roti/Rice .... 1/25 g
Curd/Dal.. 100 g/25 g
Vegetables ....1 serving (Group A)
Salad/Soup .... as desired

Bed time

Milk.. 150 ml

1200 Calories Diabetic Diet

Exchange Distribution

Food groups	*Exchange*	*Amount*	*Breakfast*	*Mid morning*	*lunch*	*Evening*	*Dinner*	*Bed Time*
Cereals	6	180 g	1	1	2	1.5	1	1.5
Pulses*	1	25 g	-	-	0.5	-	0.5	-
Milk/ Curd Toned**	4	400 ml	1.5	-	0.5	1.5	-	0.5
Fruits	2	200 g	-	1	-	1	-	-
Veg. A and B	2.5	250 g	0.5	0.5	0.5	0.5	0.5	-
Fats/Oil	3	15 ml	0.5	0.5	1.0	0.5	0.5	-

*Pulse exchange is assumed as 25 g/portion size
**Milk exchange is assumed as 100 ml/portion

Percentage Distribution of Calories

Carbohydrates .... 61 percent (180 g approx)
Proteins .... 17 percent (42 g approx)
Fats.. 22 percent (35 g approx)

Sample Menu

Breakfast

Milk/curd.. 150 ml
Bread slice/cereal/roti 2/30 g/1
Mid morning/tiffin
Roti/parantha/idli/poha .... 1/1/2/25 g + I/2 serving veg.
Fruit... 1

Lunch

Roti/Rice .... 2/50 g
Dal/Chicken .... 1/2K/75 g
Veg .... 1/2 serving
Salad... as desired

Evening
Milk... 150 ml
Cereal/Poha/Sandwich .... 1 serving/1 slice

Dinner
Roti/Rice .... 1/25 g
Dal/Chicken/Fish .... 1/2 Katori/50 g/75 g
Vegetable... 1/2 serving
Salad/Soup .... as desired
Fruit... 1

Bed Time
Milk/Cheese .... 150 ml
Biscuits (high fiber)......................... 2

1400 Calories Diabetic Diet

Exchange List

Food group	*Exchange*	*Amount (g)*	*Breakfast*	*Mid Morning*	*Lunch*	*Evening*	*Dinner*	*Bed Time*
Cereals	7	210	1.5	1.5	2	0.5	2	0.5
Pulses*	2	50	-	-	1	-	1	-
Milk/ Curd Toned**	4	400	1.5	-	0.5	1.5	-	0.5
Fruits	2	200	-	1	-	1	-	-
Veg A and B	2.5	200	-	0.5	0.5	0.5	0.5	-
Fats/Oil	2	10	-	0.5	0.5	0.5	0.5	-

*Pulse exchange is assumed as 25 g/portion size
**Milk exchange is assumed as 100 ml/portion

Percent Distribution of Calories
Carbohydrates .... 61 percent (214 g approx)
Proteins .... 17 percent (51.5 g approx)
Fats... 22 percent (30 g approx)

Sample Menu
Breakfast
Milk... 150 ml
Bread/Cereal/Roti .... 3/30 g/l

Mid Morning/Tiffin
Roti/Parantha/Idli........................... 1/1/3
*Vegetable...................................... 1/2 serving
**Fruit.. 1

Lunch

Rice/Roti 50 g/2
Dal/Curd/Chicken .... 1K/125 g/80 g
Vegetable.. 1 serving
Salad/Soup .... as desired

Evening

Milk.. 150 ml
Sprout/Bread/Besan pura/Biscuit.... 20 g/2 slices/20 g/2
Fruit.. 1

Dinner

Roti/Rice 2/50g
Dal.. 1 Katori
Vegctable.. 1/2 serving
Salad... as desired

Bed Time

Milk.. 150 ml
Biscuits-(high fiber) 2

*Vegetables from A group can be had in any amount desired
**Fruit may be selected from any low carb group

1600 Calories Diabetic Diet

Food Exchange Distribution

Food groups	*Exchange*	*Amount (g)*	*Breakfast*	*Mid Morning*	*Lunch*	*Evening*	*Dinner*	*Bed time*
Cereals	8	240	2	1	2	0.5	2	0.5
Pulses*	2	50	-	-	1	-	1	-
Milk/ Curd Toned**	5	500 ml	1.5	-	0.5	1.5	-	1.5 0.5
Fruit	2	200	-	1	-	1	-	-
Veg. A and B	2.5	250	-	0.5	1	-	1	-
Fat/Oil	3	3	0.5	0.5	1	-	1	-

*Pulse exchange is assumed as 25 g/portion size
**Milk exchange is assumed as 100 ml/portion

Percentage of Calories

Carbohydrates .... 61 percent (238.6 g approx)
Proteins .... 16 percent (58.5 g approx)
Fats.. 23 percent (40 g approx)

Sample Menu

Breakfast

Milk (toned) .... 150 ml
Parantha (stuffed)/Bread/Cereal...... 1/4/50

Mid morning

Roti/Parantha (stuffed)* 2/1
Vegetable.. 1/2 serving
Fruit.. 1

Lunch

Roti/Rice .... 2/50 g or
Roti +Rice .... 1/25 g
Dal.. 1 k
Vegetables .... 1 serving
Salad... as desired
Veg Soup .... as desired

Evening

Milk.. 150 ml
Biscuits/Cereal .... 2/10-15 g

Dinner

Roti/Rice 2/50g
Dal.. 1 katori
Vegetables .... 1 serving
Salad... as desired
Veg Soup .... as desired
Fruit.. 1

Bed time

Milk.. 150 ml
Biscuits... 2 or
Cheese Bread .... 25 g + 1 slice

*Parantha can be made without oil; stuffing with any vegetable of Group A.

1800 Calories Diabetic Diet

Exchange Distribution per Day

Food groups	*Exchange*	*Amount (g)*	*Breakfast*	*Mid Morning*	*Lunch*	*Evening*	*Dinner*	*Bed Time*
Cereals	9	270	2	2	2	0.5	2	0.5
Pulses*	2	50			1	-	1	-

Milk/Curd Toned**	5	500	1.5	-	0.5	1.5	-	1.5
Fruits	2	200	-	1	-	1	-	-
Vegetables A and B	3	300	0.5	0.5	1	-	1	-
Fats/Oil	4	20	1	0.5	1	0.5	1	-

*Pulse exchange is assumed as 25 g/portion size
**Milk exchange is assumed as 100 ml/portion

Percentage Distribution of Calories

Carbohydrtaes .... 62 percent (260 g approx)
Proteins .... 16 percent (62 g approx)
Fats .... 22 percent (45 g approx)

Sample Menu

Breakfast

Milk/Curd....................................... 150 ml
Roti/Bread/Cereal .... 2/4 slices/60 g
Vegetable.. 1/2 serving
Oil .... 0.5 ml

Mid Morning

Roti/parantha----------------------2/1
Vegetables-------------------------1/2 serving
Fruits--------------------------------1

Lunch

Roti/Rice-----------------------------2/50 g
Dal-------------------------------------1Katori
Paneer--------------------------------25g
Salad/Soup------------------------as desired

Evening

Milk--------------------------------150 ml
Biscuits-/Bread (brown)-------2/1 slice
Butter-----------------------------2.5 g

Dinner

Roti/Rice .... 2/50 g
Dal/Chicken/Fish .... 1K/80 g/100 g
Salad/Soup .... as desired
Fruit.. 1

Bed Time

Milk.. 150 ml
Biscuits.. 2

2000 Calories Diabetic Diet

Exchange Distribution per Day

Food group	*Exchange*	*Amount (g)*	*Breakfast*	*Mid Morning*	*Lunch*	*Evening*	*Dinner*	*Bed Time*
Cereals	10	300	2	1.5	3	1	3	0.5
Pulses*	3	75	-	0.5		0.5	1 1	-
Milk/ Curd Toned**	5	500	1.5	-	0.5	1.5	-	1.5
Fruits	2	200	-	1	-	1	-	-
Veg A and B	3	300	0.25	1.5	1	0.25	1	-
Fats/Oil	4	20	1.0	0.5	1	0.5	1	-

*Pulse is assumed as 25 g/portion size
**Milk is assumed as 100 ml/portion

Percentage Distribution of Calories

Carbohydrtaes .... 62 percent (295 g approx)
Proteins .... 16 percent (71.5 g approx)
Fats... 22 percent (46.2 g approx)

Sample Menu

Breakfast

Milk/Curd... 250 ml
Roti*/Bread/Cereal .... 2/4 slices/60 g
Vegetables .... 1/2 serving (Group A)

Mid morning

Roti/Parantha*................................. 2/1
Vegetable... 1/2 serving (Group A)
Fruit.. 1 (low carb)

Lunch

Roti/Rice .... 3/75 g
Dal/Chicken/Fish .... 1 katori/80 g/100 g

Evening

Milk.. 250 ml
Biscuits/Sandwich........................... 3/2 slices
Fruit** .... 1 (low carb)

Dinner

Roti/Rice .... 3/75 g
Dal/Chicken/Fish .... 1 katori/80 g/100 g
Vegetables .... 1 serving
Salad/Soup .... as desired

*Roti/parantha may be made of wheat and gram flour in 2:1 ratio.
**Fruit can be had at any convenient time of the day.

REFERENCES

1. Davies JL, Kawaguchi Y, Bennet ST, et al. A genome wide search for human type 1 diabetes susceptible genes. Nature, 1994;371:130-6.
2. Dahlquist G. Environmental risk factors in human Type 1 diabetes- an epidemiological perspective. Diabetes Metab. Rev. 1995;11:37-46.
3. Dahlquist GG, Blom LG, Persson lA, Sandstorm AM, Wall SGL. Dietary factors and the risk of developing insulin dependent diabetes in childhood. BMJ, 1990;1300:1302-6.
4. Verge CF, Howard NJ, Irving L, Simpson JM, Mackerras D, Silinik M. Environmental factors in childhood IDDM. Diabetes Care. 1994;17: 1381-9.
5. Scott FW, Cow's milk intake and insulin dependent diabetes: is there a relationship? Am J Clin Nutr 1990;51:489-91.
6. Savilhatti E, Akaerblom HK, Tainio VM, Koskimies S. Children with newly diagnosed insulin dependent diabetes mellitus have increased levels of cow's milk antibodies. Diabetes Res 1998;137-40.
7. Kostraba JN, Cruickshanks KJ, Lawler-Heavner J, et al. Early exposure to cow's milk and solid foods in infancy, genetic predisposition and risk of IDDM. Diabetes 1993;42:282-95.
8. Sandro Muntoni, Pierluigi Cucco, Gabriella Aru, Francesso Cucco, Sergio Muntoni. Nutritional factors and worldwide incidence of childhood type 1 diabetes. Am J Clin Nutr 2000;71:1525-9.
9. Donmer G, Thoelka H, Mohnike A, Schneider H. High food supply in perinatal life appears to favour the development of insulin treated diabetes mellitus (ITM) in later life. Exp Clin Endocrinol 1985;85:1-6.
10. Johansson C, Samvelsson U, Ludvisgson J. A high weight gain early in life is associated with an increased risk of type 1 (insulin dependent) diabetes mellitus. Diabetologia 1994;34:91-4.
11. Borch-Johnsen K, Mandrip-Poulsen T, Zachau-Christainsen B, Joner G, Christy M, Kastrip K, Nerup J. Relation between breastfeeding and incidence of rates of insulin dependent diabetes mellitus. Lancet 1984;1083-86.
12. Ayer EJ, Hamman RF, gay EC, Lezatte DC, Savitz DA, Kingensmith GJ: Reduced risk of IDDM among breastfed children: The Colorado IDDM Registry. Diabetes 1998;37:1625-32.

13. Kyvik Ko, Green A, Svendsen A, Montensen K. Breastfeeding and the development of type 1 diabetes mellitus. Diabetes Med 1992;223-35.
14. Ingersoll GM, Orr D, Herrold AJ, Golden MP. Cognitive maturity and self management in adolescents with insulin dependent diabetes mellitus. J Pediatr 1986;108:620-3.
15. American Diabetes Association. Diagnosis and classification of diabetes mellitus (Position Statement). Diabetes Care 2004;27 (Suppl 1): S5-S10.
16. Scibili J, Finegold D, Dorman J, Becker D, Drash A. Why do children with diabetes die? Acta Endocrinol Suppl (Copenh) 1986;279:326-33.
17. Talbot JM, Fischer KD. The need for special foods and sugar substitutes by individuals with diabetes mellitus. Diabetes Care 1978;1: 231-40.
18. Belton NR, Farquhar JW, Diabetes mellitus. In: Chemical Pathology and the Sick Child (Clayton BE, Round JM (Eds)). 1984;pp265-95; Oxford: Blackwell Scientific Publications.
19. American Diabetic Assoc. Statement, Care of children and Adolescents with Type 1 Diabetes. Janet Silverstein, Georgeanna Klingensmith, Kenneth Copeland etal. Diabetes Care 2005, Vol 28, No.1, Jan.
20. Randecker GA, Smiciklas-Wright H, Mc Kenzie JM, et al. The dietary intake of children with insulin dependent diabetes mellitus. Diabetes Care 1996;19:1370-74.
21. American Academy of Pediatrics. National Cholesterol Education Program Report of the Expert Panel on Blood Cholesterol Levels in Children and Adolescents, Pediatrics 1992;89:525-84.
22. Report of the Nutrition Sub Committee of the Medical Advisory Committee of the British Diabetic Association; Dietary Recommendations for diabetics for the 1980s. Human Nutr: Appl Nutr, 1982;36A:378-94.
23. Nutrition Sub Committee of the Professional Advisory Committee of the British Diab Assoc. Dietary Recommendations for children and adolescents with diabetes. Diabetic Medicine,1989;6:537-47.
24. American Diabetic Association. Recommendations and principles for individuals with diabetes mellitus: 1986, Diabetes care 1987;10:126-32.
25. Simpson RW, Mann JI, Eaton J, et al. High carbohydrate diets and insulin dependent diabetics. BMJ 1979;2:523-5.
26. Simpson RW, Mann JI, Eaton J, et al. Improved glucose control in maturity onset diabetes treated with high carbohydrate modified fat diet. BMJ 1979;1:1753-6.
27. Vanessa Shaw, Margaret Lawson. Diabetes Mellitus. In: Clinical Pediatric Nutrition 2nd ed Blackwell Publishers pg. 127-135.
28. Wolfsdorf JI, Quinn M. Diabetes Mellitus. In: Nutrition in Pediatrics, Basic Science and Clinical Applications. Walker WA, Watkins JB (Eds). 1997 BC Decker Inc. Publishers Hamilton. London.
29. Gopalan C, Rama Sastri BV, Balasubramanian SC. Nutritive Values of Indian Foods. National Institute of Nutrition, ICMR, Hyderabad.

30. Wolever TM, Hanad S, Chiasson JL, Josse RG, et al. Day to day consistency in amount and source of carbohydrate associated with improved blood glucose control in Type 1 diabetes. J Am Coll Nutr 1999;18:242-7.
31. Diabetes Care and Education Dietetic Practice Group of the ADA. Meal Planning Approaches for Diabetes Management. 2nd ed. Alexandria, VA: American Dietetics Association; 1994:3.
32. Jenkins DJA, Wolever TMS, Taylor RH, et al. Glycemic index of foods: A physiological basis for carbohydrate exchange. Am. J Clin Nutr 1981; 34:362-6.
33. Jenkins DJA, Taylor RH, Wolever TMS. The diabetic diet, dietary carbohydrate and differences in digestibility. Diabetologia 1982;23:477-84.
34. Position Statement, American Diabetic Assoc. Nutrition recommendations and principles for people with diabetes mellitus. Diabetes Care 1994;17:519-22.
35. Raghuram TC, Swaran Pasricha, Sharma RD. Diet and Diabetes, National Institute of Nutrition, ICMR, Hyderabad, 1998.
36. Jenkins DJA, Wolevar TMS, Leads AR, et al. Dietary fibers, fiber analogues and glucose intolerance: Importance of viscosity. BMJ 1978;1: 1392-4.
37. Farhath Khanum, Swamy S, Sudarshana Krishna KR, Sanathanam K, Viswanathan KR. Dietary fiber content of common fresh and cooked vegetables consumed in India. Plant Foods for Human Nutrition 2000;55:207-18.
38. National Cholesterol Education Program. Report of the Expert Panel on Blood Cholesterol Levels in children and Adolescents. Pediatrics 1992; 89 (Suppl): 525-84.
39. Bantle JP, Laine DC, castle GW, et al. Post prandial glucose and insulin responses to meals containing different carbohydrates in normal and diabetic subjects. N Eng J Med 1983;309:7-12.
40. Abraira C, Derler J. Large variations of sucrose in constant carbohydrate diets in Type II diabetes. Am J Med 1988;84:193-200.
41. Wise JE, Keim KS, Huisinga LJ, William PA. Effect of sucrose containing snacks on blood glucose control. Diabetes Care 1989;12:423-6.
42. Council on Scientific affairs. Aspartame review of safety issues. JAMA 1985;254:400-2.
43. Drash A. The child, the adolescent and the diabetes control and complications trial. Dibetes Cre. 1993;16:1515-6.
44. Chalmers KH. Diabetes In: Handbook of Pediatric Nutrition 2nd ed. Patricia Queen Samour, Kathy King Helm and Carol E. Lang (2004), Jones and Bartlett Publishers, Massachusetts pp 425-51.

Chapter 12 Dietary Management in Hypoglycemia

If hyperglycemia is a problem of serious consequences, hypoglycemia too is equally significant with regards to normal growth and development of a child. Consequences of hypoglycemia are permanent damage to the central nervous system (CNS), particularly in infants under six months and hence corrective dietary measures need to be taken as soon as the problem is diagnosed.

Hypoglycemia may be asymptomatic or could be associated with features of listlessness, apathy, irritability, pallor, sweating, weakness, hunger, headache, nausea, mental confusion, convulsions and coma. It could vary considerably in their type of presentation and the mechanisms involved. In general the main types of hypoglycemia of dietary interest are:

- Glycogen Storage Disease Type I (Glucose-6-phosphatase deficiency)
- Glycogen Storage Disease Type III and VI (Debrancher enzyme deficiency)
- Leucine Sensitive Hypoglycemia.

GLYCOGEN STORAGE DISEASE TYPE I (GLUCOSE-6-PHOSPHATASE DEFICIENCY)

As we know glycogen is the body's major carbohydrate reserve consisting of glucose molecules linked together into a branched chain. It is synthesized in the liver from glucose and is dependent on adequate glucose-6-phospatase activity. A regular maintenance level of glucose in the blood is required continuously and is essential for normal growth and development.

In this disorder due to the deficiency of the enzyme glucose-6-phosphatase, glucose is not released into the circulation and therefore a regular supply of it has to be ensured through dietary source, mainly carbohydrates. In the absence of continuous supply of dietary carbohydrates, serious consequences like growth retardation, hyperlipidemia and raised plasma uric acid can occur. Regular administration of carbohydrates to maintain normal blood glucose levels helps prevent secondary features of metabolic acidosis and maintain growth.[1]

Management of these children in infancy involves continuous IV glucose to maintain normoglycemia. However, such a regimen cannot be continued indefinitely over a long period. Therefore after the initial maintenance phase, oral carbohydrate can be started to provide 0.5 g carbohydrate/kg per hour in infancy and gradually decreasing to 0.1 g carbohydrate per hour in older children. This dose can be provided in the form of glucose polymers (15-25 percent solution) as per requirements based on age. Overnight nasogastrofeeding is advisable to maintain glucose levels during the night, while at day time 2-3 hourly glucose drinks can be given orally. However, care should be taken in overnight feeding to avoid risk of any accidental pulling or displacement of the tube or any leaks.

In older children a mixed home based diet with high source of carbohydrate is preferable at 2-3 hours intervals as absorption gets slower with oral feeds. The amount of carbohydrates calculated should be adequate to maintain normal blood glucose levels.

Another simple and established way of ensuring sustained release of glucose and thus avert any likelihood of hypoglycemia (especially during the night), is ingestion of uncooked starch which has been very beneficial in older children. When given orally, raw corn starch is slowly hydrolysed by pancreatic amylase and intestinal glucoamylase to provide a steady supply of exogenous glucose throughout the dosing interval, thereby preventing hypoglycemia. Cornstarch therapy was reported to be less effective in infants whose secretion of pancreatic amylase may be insufficient to hydrolyse the cornstarch granules.[2] Compared with nocturnal intragastric feeding cornstarch therapy is less invasive, more economical and simpler to administer. These factors serve to increase patient compliance with corn starch therapy.[3] Studies have shown best results with uncooked cornstarch mixed with water at room temperature. A dose of 1-2 g/kg body weight given twice daily, at night time and at lunch allows for a greater flexibility of glucose ingestion by daytime. However, this regimen is not suitable for infants, as the pancreatic amylase required to digest raw starch is absent or negligible in the newborn and reaches adult levels at 2-4 years of age. For newborns and infants, it is preferable to give nocturnal infusions and frequent feeds.[4]

The dose of raw cornstarch varies from one child to another and must be assessed individually. Care must be taken that children with this problem should not be allowed to remain fasting and any infections treated promptly. It has been proposed by authors that uncooked cornstarch should be postponed till pubertal growth spurt of the child has been attained.[3]

The benefit of using cornstarch as compared to continuous nocturnal glucose feeding has been reported by some workers who observed better social acceptance by patients and caregivers. The only flaw reported by them is the need to take it every 6 hours which generally interrupted the sleep of the children. Moreover, they also reported that although cornstarch mixed with water did not maintain normoglycemia in infants,[5] but some other studies also showed that when it was mixed with milk or curd and given every 4 hourly could benefit young infants as young as 8 months old.[6]

Large quantities of lactose and sucrose from which galactose and fructose are most commonly derived, should be avoided in young children to avoid the risk of metabolic acidosis. Metabolic acidosis occurs due to failure of conversion of galactose and fructose to glucose, resulting in production of lactate.

Glucose Polymers

Glucose polymers are commercially available in the Western market as polycose glucose polymers. These are easily digestible source of carbohydrate calories for use when additional carbohydrate calories are required, especially in electrolytes or fat restricted diets. These are derived from controlled hydrolysis of cornstarch. The main features of these polymers are:

- Rapid absorption (peak glucose response in 30 minutes)
- Longer glucose polymers reduce osmolality, thus reducing risk of osmotic diarrhea
- These have a low renal solute
- Mix easily with food and beverage
- Minimal sweeteners to enhance acceptance
- Lactose and gluten free.

The main criterion for preparing a diet for children with type I glycogen storage disease is summarized as follows:

- 0.5 g/kg of carbohydrates per hour to be initiated as 1-2 hourly oral drinks by day and as overnight continuous nasogastric drip. To decrease to 0.01 g/kg /hr in older children
- Milk should be minimal or avoided initially and substituted by glucose or starch or glucose polymers, if available
- Vegetable oils and polyunsaturated fatty acids are preferable to saturated fats
- Honey should be avoided due to the high content of fructose

- Artificial sweeteners like sorbitol or fructose based should be avoided
- Fruits to be avoided due to their high fructose content
- Medicines containing sorbitol, lactose or sucrose should be avoided
- All vegetables may be permitted
- All cereals without sugar may be allowed
- Diet should be adequate in all other nutrients as per the RDA for individual age.

GLYCOGEN STORAGE DISEASE TYPES III AND VI (DEBRANCHER ENZYME DEFICIENCY)

These types of glycogen storage disease also manifest features of hypoglycemia, hepatomegaly, growth failure and hyperglycemia, but in a milder form as compared to the Type I. In this condition glycogen cannot be broken down to release glucose, thereby favouring conditions of starvation as a result of hypoglycemia.[1] But plasma glucose levels can be maintained through other pathways since the metabolism of amino acids, galactose and fructose are not affected. Therefore there is a wider choice of carbohydrates from dietary source. To avoid hypoglycemia, fasting is advised against and a high protein diet with frequent meals and or drinks should be continuously offered. A protein and starch based snack is advisable to be given at bed time to avoid feeding in the middle of the night.

A normal diet with high protein sources, low fats preferably polyunsaturated type and moderate carbohydrates is ideal for patients with these types of storage disorders. A comparison between the two types of storage disorders is summarized in Table 12.1.[1]

The use of uncooked starch gas also been advocated in Type III glycogen storage disorders with beneficial results.[7, 8] Experience of other workers has suggested that oral cornstarch can be effective as an initial therapy as well as a maintainenance therapy for children with GSD III. Besides, the clinical response in their patients suggested that cornstarch therapy may be as effective as other proposed forms of treatment for GSD III, like protein supplementation or nasogastric formula infusion. However, it was also cautioned that poor linear growth velocity should be considered as an indication of this treatment of patients with GSD III.[9]

LEUCINE SENSITIVE HYPOGLYCEMIA

This condition is a very rare disorder which involves leucine sensitivity. It manifests in the form of acute fall in blood sugars in certain infants and

Table 12.1: Summary of diets in hepatic glycogen storage diseases

Type I *Glucose-6-phosphatase deficiency*	*Types III and VI* *Debrancher enzyme deficiency*
Carbohydrates: Glucose, glucose polymers And starch providing 50-70 percent energy Limit galactose, fructose, lactose and Sucrose in diet of young children Avoid sorbitol	All carbohydrates esp. starch/slow release
Protein: Normal intake for all ages	High protein intake up to twice the normal requirement for all ages.
Fat: Preferably polyunsaturated	Preferably polyunsaturated
Frequency: Young children-overnight	Late night protein rich carbohydrate glucose as continuous drip and 1-2 supper or overnight drinks.
Hourly drinks by day; older children-	Frequent meals and drinks uncooked starch

Source: Francis DEM, Diets in Hypoglycemia, In: Diets for sick children pp 348-56

young children. The onset is generally observed in the first year of life and if the condition goes undetected, it may also lead to mental retardation and neurological symptoms. There is no abnormality in the metabolism of leucine but it is considered that there may be an accumulation of excess leucine in the blood. A high protein diet generally triggers the situation.

Management of the condition involves immediate administration of glucose for brain metabolism either orally or intravenously. It is speculated that this condition may disappear by age of 4-6 years.[10] Drugs like diazoxide with or without diet is considered to be effective in treating the condition. Dietary treatment involves limiting of leucine rich diets which can be done by selecting infant formulae which are modified for their protein content with reduced leucine composition. As for any other form of hypoglycemia it is advised that frequent feeding of the child may be continued and keep a watch on any signs of hypoglycemia. Some children may require as much as 1 g of carbohydrate for each 5 mg of leucine to prevent hypoglycemia, necessitating 4-6 hourly feeds daily and boosting up with carbohydrate drinks during the night time too. In acute illness when the child is unable to ingest adequate amounts, drinks of 15-20 g carbohydrates should be offered at frequent intervals.

KETOTIC HYPOGLYCEMIA

This type of hypoglycemia occurs more frequently among the male children in the toddler age group. Symptoms include apathy, listlessness, convulsions and coma, which revert with ingestion of food. Management involves avoiding long duration of fasting and feeding frequently. Dietary carbohydrate source should be higher and spaced out during the day. However excess of fats and fried foods should be avoided. In conditions when the child is sick and refuses to eat, carbohydrate based drinks can be offered every 2-3 hourly over the day to avoid long hours of fasting. Any leftover food should be re served after a small interval or be replaced by any carbohydrate based drink, e.g. 15 or 20 g of carbohydrate increasing to 40-50 g in the older age group.[1] (See Table 11.5 Chapter 11, for CHO exchange).

It is advisable to counsel parents to test for ketones in the urine and if positive, to give carbohydrate drinks as explained above along with sodium bicarbonate.

REFERENCES

1. Francis DEM. Diets in hypoglycemia In: Diets for sick children pp 348-56; 4th Edition. Blackwell Scientific Publications 1987.
2. Chen YT, Cornblath M, Sidbury JB. Cornstarch therapy in Type I glycogen storage disease. N Engl J Med 1984;310:171-5.
3. Borowitz SM, Greene HL. Cornstarch therapy in a patient with Type I glycogen storage disease. J Pediatr Gastroenterol Nutr 1987;6:631-4.
4. Smit GPA, Berger R, Potasnick R, Moses SW and Fernandes J. The dietary treatment of Type I glycogen storage disease with slow release carbohydrate. Pediatr Res. 1984;18(9):879-81.
5. Chen YT, Bazzare CH, Lee MM, Sidbury JB and Coleman RA. Type I glycogen storage disease: Nine years of management with cornstarch. Eur J Pediatr 1993, 152 (Suppl):556-9.
6. Wolfsderf JI, Keller RJ, LandyH, Crigler JF, et al. Glucose therapy for glycogenolysis Type I in infants: Comparison of intermittent uncooked cornstarch and continuous overnight glucose feedings. J Pediatr 1990; 117:384-91.
7. Gremse CS, Bucuvalas JC, Balistrerri WF. Efficacy of cornstarch therapy in Type III glycogen storage disease. Am J Clin Nutr 1990,52:671-4.
8. Ullrich K, Schmitt H, Van Teefelen Heithoff A. Glycogen storage disease Type I and III and pyruvate carbohydrate deficiency: Results of long-term treatment and uncooked corn starch. *Acta Pediatr Scand.* 1988;77:531-6.
9. Wolfsdorf JI, Rudlin CR and Crigler JF Jr. Physical growth and development of children with Type I glycogen storage: Comparison of the effects of long-term use of dextrose and uncooked starch. Am J Clin Nutr 1990;52:1051-7.
10. WB Saunders, Cornblath M and Schwartz R. In: Disorders of Carbohydrate Metabolism in Infancy (Vol. III in the series- Major Problems of Clinic Pediatrics). 2nd edition (Ed. Schaffer AI).1976, philadelphia: pp231-93.

Chapter 13

The Ketogenic Diet in Management of Epilepsy

The treatment of epilepsy has been described since the era of Hippocrates in 400 BC,[1] when it was considered as a prophetic curse. He refuted this belief and advocated 'purging and fasting' as a cure for the disease. Detoxification method was also used by earlier workers in 1911 by Guelpa and Marie[2] by reducing vegan diet and fasting and purging.

HISTORY OF KETOGENIC DIET (KD)

In 1920, Russel Wilder at Mayo Clinic proposed that the benefits of fasting would be obtained by producing high levels of ketones in the body (ketonemia) through excess of fat and lack of carbohydrates. This led to the coining of the new term 'ketogenic diet'. In 1921, Geylin first reported about fasting as an alternative treatment to anti epileptic drugs (AED) for controlling intractable seizures. In the 26 patients who were fasted for 15-25 days, 18 of his patients showed marked improvement. This was attributed to a neutralization of the deleterious effects of toxins from the Peyer's patches in the intestines.[2]

Wilder's colleague pediatrician Myne Peterman later formulated the 'classic diet' with a ratio of 1 g of protein per kg body weight and 10-15 g carbohydrates (CHO)/day and the balance calories to be obtained from fat. This diet was seemingly supposed to mimic the metabolic effects of fasting. This was akin to the 4:1 ratio keto diet used today.

In 1938, Dr. Merritt and Petermann discovered dilantin and subsequently in 1939, phenytoin became the drug of choice in the management of epilepsy. Then followed an advent of a series of AEDs like carbamazepine in 1950s, clonazepam in 1974, sodium valporate in 1978 and clobazam in 1979. As a result fewer children were placed on KD, leading to a steady decline in the use of KD. In 1971, Dr. Huttenlocher introduced the MCT diet in an attempt to retain the beneficial effect which was less restrictive and easier to administer. This diet was found to be too rigid, too unpalatable and difficult to prepare and maintain.[3]

THE STORY OF CHARLIE

Charlie was a young boy of 2 years and half, who first developed seizures on March 11, 1993, which could not be controlled and by 1994, he had as many as 100 seizures a day. None of the drugs worked for him and it was then that his father Jim Abraham, a TV producer heard of John Hopkins Hospital and the KD. Charlie was put on KD and within a few days, he stopped having seizures. He continued on this diet for 2 years, remaining totally seizure free and then stopped. Within a few days seizures again recurred and he was back on KD. Subsequently, he became seizure free and went off the diet and medication for many years. It was then that Jim started the 'Charlie Foundation. He produced a video about Charlie's story and sent it to every pediatric neurologist in the US. In 1955, Charlie Foundation started the first multicentric study on KD.[4] In 1997, he produced a movie 'First do no harm', starring Meryl Streep and Millicent Kelly, a dietician at John Hopkins Hospital.

MECHANISM OF ACTION OF KD

The KD is a diet with high fat content, which causes conversion of fats to ketones, which are further utilized for energy instead of glucose. This diet allows incomplete oxidation of fatty acids by the liver resulting in the accumulation of ketone bodies in urine and blood. The body uses these ketones instead of glucose as a source of energy. When carbohydrates are deprived to the body by prolonged fasting, the body begins to utilize fats and proteins for fuel. As fats are oxidized for energy, they are not oxidized completely thereby resulting in a build-up of residues or waste products of acetone and ketone bodies. These ketone bodies build-up in the blood and spill over into the urine, resulting in a state of ketosis. This has an anticonvulsant effect, thereby inhibiting seizures.[4] Others put forth the theory that certain changes occur at the neurotransmitter level which improves cerebral energy.[5]

While on a ketogenic diet, the body does not solely rely on stored fat and ketones as the primary fuel source. It will also rely on dietary fats. This is the major difference between starvation and ketogenesis. This is also why one cannot consume unlimited calories on a ketogenic diet and expect to lose weight. The body will use dietary fats as a primary fuel source along with the subsequent ketone bodies from oxidation of dietary fats and then will use adipose, only if the calories are maintained at a level below that required to maintain body weight. If calories are maintained at suboptimal level on KD, the body is forced to begin lipolysis. This becomes the primary energy source with other physiological mechanisms stepping-up to allow normal and efficient functioning while on KD.[6]

SELECTION OF PATIENTS FOR KETOGENIC DIET

Type of Epilepsy

The response to KD is largely based on the type of seizure of childhood, like myoclonic, where good response has been reported.[7] Those with tonic clonic (grand mal) epilepsy may be helped, but in other types of seizures this diet may not be effective. Children with refractory epilepsy were found to benefit more with the diet as compared to any alternative anticonvulsant drug.[7]

For patients who benefit, half will achieve a seizure reduction within 5 days. If the diet starts with an initial fast of 1-2 days, three, fourths achieve a seizure reduction within a fortnight and 90 percent achieve reduction within 23 days. If the diet does not begin with a fast, the time achieved for about 50 percent of the children could be longer, but the long-term seizure rates are unaffected. Since fasting increases the risk of acidosis and hypoglycemia, it is recommended only in some medical emergency. A carbohydrate washout regimen is a better alternative before initiating KD. If no improvement is seen within 2 months, it indicates failure of the diet.[8]

Age of the Patient

Ketogenic diet has been found to be most effective in children between ages 2-5 years old. These children become ketotic soon and maintain adequate levels of ketosis with the diet. The diet seems to get less effective with each progressive year and by adolescence, is rarely found to be successful.[9] On the other hand very young children rarely produce ketosis and hence not indicated.[10] Infants are at greatest risk from nutritional deficiencies of the dietary regimen and therefore should be avoided in this age group.

Motivation/Compliance

The KD can be successful and adhered to only if there is a complete rapport between the parents and the patients and the dietetic and metabolic team. If the diet is not complied with rigidly, the ketotic effect disappears thus nullifying the benefit effect of going through the whole exercise. Accidental lapse or pilfering of carbohydrates based diet, if taken at any point even in minute amounts can negate the ketosis, thereby bringing back the seizures which may falsely implicate failure of the diet.

Failure of AEDs

KD is initiated only after at least 2-3 medicines have failed, as it is not very easy to administer and maintain on this diet. Moreover, the diet is comparatively rigid and demands lifestyle changes.

Literacy and Socioeconomic Factor

Following a KD involves some expenditure in terms of dietary products to be procured, which need to be labeled for all the nutritive values. This therapy involves measuring urine ketones daily to ensure adequate ketosis and this requires use of keto diastix to measure ketosis. These diastix are not very cheap and regular use entails recurrent expenditure. It may not be financially possible for families with limited resources. Literacy level of parents/care givers too is crucial since the diet maintenance requires careful weighing of all ingredients and reading all food labels before preparing the diet.

Other Factors

Patients with infantile spasms who respond poorly to medication should also be considered for KD. According to Dr. Nathan, since there is 90 percent improvement in children with infantile spasm on KD, it is recommended to initiate this diet as first line of treatment.[11] Children who are retarded, or are fed by gastrostomy tube or on Ryle's tube, may also be suitable candidates for KD, as it is easier to use and be more effective than trying medications.

INITIATING KETOGENIC DIET

Initiating ketogenic diet involves 4 phases as follows:[11]

Phase 1

Pre Diet Counseling: Before a patient is put on KD, it is very important that the parents be counseled regarding all the details of the therapy and need to be explained the rationale behind this mode of therapy in a scientific way:

- It has to be impressed upon them that they should not expect miracles from the therapy. However, they can be reassured regarding the goal of this type of management, even though results may be appreciated not before 4-6 weeks of initializing the diet
- The importance of actually weighing the food ingredients and use of only instructed food items in prescribed portions should be explained and impressed upon them for the therapy to be successful. If possible,

a list of recipes and their demonstration of preparing them will create a greater impact

- Demonstration of urine testing for ketones needs to be done and a ketone chart should be maintained. This helps both parents and the dietician and the keto team to obtain a fair feedback of the efficacy of the diet
- Parents need to understand that the yardstick of success of the diet is gauged by reduction/control of seizures
- Reduction of AEDs comes secondary and may be found in about 30 percent, another 30 percent may be totally free of seizures while the rest 40 percent may not show any reduction
- Most children may show generalized mental alertness and increase in intelligence
- Care givers/parents need to be explained regarding the history of dietary management, which can help them adhere and comply strictly to the diet
- All medications have to be sugar free, even to the extent of the tooth paste used, which can contain some sugar
- Sugar free toothpastes like Vicco or Meswak should be used only
- While using IV fluids, only saline should be used instead of dextrose based
- Keto diets may be with held for sometime during periods of acute illness or infections.

Initializing of the KD: Managing a child with KD requires the following steps:

1. ***Personal history:*** This includes details relating to the patients contacts, family physician, family members at home, grandparents and other members in a joint family, who also need to be counseled regarding the significance of the KD, meticulous planning and execution of the diet.
2. ***Anthropometry:*** Recording of the weight and height of the patient is the primary step before planning a KD, since the calories fixed are based upon the ideal body weight (IBW) and involves a formula using both parameters. However, height recording may be problem in children with presence of spaticity and contactures.
3. ***Medical history:*** History regarding any preexisting problems of allergies has to be considered, other chronic ailments like asthma, diabetes mellitus, tuberous sclerosis should be also accounted for while planning the diet. Other AEDs prescribed need to be recorded.
4. ***Diet history:*** While planning a diet for the child, it is worthwhile to extract certain details of the eating patterns likes/dislikes, the number

of meals taken over the day, preferences, and religious issues, e.g. vegetarian or nonvegetarian and any other relevant ethnic background information.

5. ***Investigations:*** Some common investigations required are serum proteins, CBC, Lipid profile, serum electrolytes, serum calcium, uric acid, serum creatinine, blood sugars, and liver enzymes along with blood for gas values. EEG and physcometric examinations need to be done at the beginning and once annually thereafter.

Phase 2

Carbohydrate Wash Out or Pre Keto Diet: In the earlier days before initializing the KD, the patient was made to fast for 1-2 days to enable to produce ketosis easily. But gradually the practice of fasting was rarely followed and instead a carbohydrate wash out is administered to achieve a ketosis of 4+ within 3-4 days. The advantage of this diet is that it does not require any exact weighing of food or fixing timings of meals. The major constituents of this diet are fats and proteins and negligible carbohydrates. A list of foods that can be given during the carbohydrate wash out phase are listed in Table 13.1.

Certain points need to be borne in mind while following a CHO wash out diet like:

- Offer small frequent feeds
- Check urine ketones
- Free foods to be given in between like sugar free jelly, sugar free sherbet
- Offer water unrestricted
- No calculations or weighing of foods needed
- Follow a diet for a minimum of 2-3 days to achieve 4+ ketones
- No hospitalization required.

Prerequisite of a Ketogenic Diet: Before the actual KD is initiated, during the CHO wash out phase, parents are advised to procure the following items to actually prepare and monitor the diet:

- Digital weighing scale with ± 1 g accuracy
- Other kitchen items like measuring cups, glass, spoons, airtight containers, nonstick pan, fiber spatula rubber and wooden spatula
- Urine keto diastics for measuring ketones.

Phase 3

Once the ketone levels of 4+ are achieved on a CHO wash out diet, or even if not and on the diet for at least 3-4 days, the ketogenic diet is

Table 13.1: Foods allowed and restricted in CHO wash out phase

Not allowed	*Allowed moderately*	*Allowed liberally*
All cereals/pulses: Chapati, rice, suji, dals Gram flour, corn flour	Tomato, cucumber–5 g	All nonveg. foods: Chicken, fish, eggs, home-made mayonnaise
Sugar and sweets: All sweets, honey, jaggery, all bakery products	Amul/Britannia cheese/paneer–1 cube	All soya products: Soya flour, soya dal, soya rawa, soya granules, soya milk (Godrej-Sofit/Natural Staeta)
All processed foods, aspartame, sugar free tabs.	Amul cream – 50 g	Beverages-water, plain soda (color, essence, sugar free natura tab)
Vegetables-all root vegetables Fruits-Banana, mangoes, chikkoo	Almonds, walnuts, groundnuts – 5	Fats and oils- butter, ghee
Medicines-syrups or any sugar coated pills, toothpaste, IV dextrose		Sugar free toothpaste-Vicco/Meswak, IV Saline

calculated and planned by the dietician. The ratio of the keto diet has to be fixed, i.e. 2:1 or 3:1 or 4:1 depending upon the age, severity of seizures, etc. and then the ideal body weight (IBW) for the child is derived from his height and weight.

Diet Calculations

The steps involved in the calculations are as follows:

a. To begin with the IBW is derived for the given child which works out to be 50th centile of IBW-50th centile of height X actual height.
b. The calories required are then derived which should be 75 percent of the RDA for the given child as per his age (Table 17.2).
c. Next the keto ratio has to be decided, which is the ratio of grams of fat to the sum of grams of carbohydrate and proteins, e.g. 2:1, 3:1 or 4:1. In a ratio of 2:1, it implies that 2 g of fat to 1 g of protein and carbohydrates combined. For instance 2×9 (cals.per g from fat) = 18 and 1x4 (cals. per g from carbohydrate and protein), i.e. $18 + 4 = 22$. So, the Dietary Unit Composition (DUC) = 22.
d. Next Dietary Unit Quotient (DUQ) is calculated as Calories-DUC
e. **Fat Allowance** = DUQ × 2 (keto ratio)
f. CHO +Protein allowance (C+P)= DUQ × 1 (C+P ratio)
g. **Protein Allowance:** This is calculated for a given age group based on the RDA (see Table 17.3) which may range from 1-1.5 g/Kg/d.

h. **CHO allowance = C+P –P**

i. **Meal Order:** This is the number of meals the child would consume per day, e.g. 4, 5 or 6. meals/day. This number divided by the total fats, carbohydrates and protein allowance is the per meal distribution for fats, carbohydrates and proteins.

PLANNING OF RECIPES

It is important that each recipe is calculated based on the derived fat, carbohydrate and protein for that specific patient. For this, the dietician needs to be aware of and have a list of all commercial food products available locally, so as to be able to calculate the exact values. A table of nutritive values of different foods per 100 grams should be at hand for ready reference.[12] Knowledge of all the locally available commercial foods is essential, which can be used in various recipes and parents need to be encourage to use those products only for preparing the KD. Vegetables and fruits are divided into A and B groups depending upon their carbohydrate content as given in Tables 13.2A and B.[12] There are some free foods which can be given to the child in unrestricted amount and any time of the day. These are:

- Sugar free, flavored sherbet, juices (sugar free should be sucrolose based only, e.g. naturla gold
- Sugar free jelly, ice candy
- Gelatin, jelly
- Plain soda

The food groups that can be given in a ketogenic diet are as listed in Table 13.3.

Considerations or Special Categories of Patients

A. ***Overweight children:*** In case of overweight children, it is recommended to reduce and achieve desirable weight, which can be done by reducing 100 calories from the calculated 75 percent of the RDA for the given age group. It is essential that the child burns the excess body weight. A brief diet history can give an idea of the pre diet intake. The activity level of the child also will determine the required calories.

B. ***Underweight children:*** In case of underweight children, if calories are inadequate, there is risk of the proteins being utilized for energy, therefore it is recommended to add 100 calories to the derived 75 percent of the RDA for the given child.

C. ***Fluid allowance:*** The fluid allowance for a child on KD is generally 1 ml/cal.

Table 13.2A: Food exchange list for vegetables*

Vegetable A Group (4 percent CHO)–20 g	*Vegetable B Group (8 percent CHO)–10 g*
Amaranth (Chaulai), Bitter gourd, bottle gourd, brinjal, capsicum, cucumber, green papaya, tomato, parwal, French beans, ridge gourd, snake gourd, spinach, tinda, white radis	Onions, broad beans, cauliflower, cluster beans, cabbage, carrots, fenugreek

*Veg. Group B =1/2 of Veg. Group A
Ref. (12) ICMR values

Table 13.2B: Food exchange list for fruits*

Fruit A (10 percent CHO)–15 g	*B (15 percent CHO) – 10 g*
Figs, guava, sweet lime (mausambi), muskmelon, watermrlon, orange ripe, pears, papaya, plums, raspberry, strawberry, rose apple (jambool)	Amla, apple, ramphal, cashew fruit, red cherries, grapes (blue and green), lichi, mango ripe, pomegranate (anar), prunes.

*Fruit B = 2/3rd of Fruit A
Ref. (12) ICMR values

Table 13.3: List of foods to be given in a ketogenic diet

	Foods restricted	*Foods unrestricted*
STOP (Carbohydrate source)	Given in less amounts (CHO foods)	Vegetables, fruits, cereals, pulses, milk, some spices
LOOK (Fats and Proteins)	Given in liberal amounts (fats and protein foods)	Fats, oils, cheese, paneer, cream, chicken, fish, egg, soya products
GO (Free)	Free Foods	Sugar free, jelly, zero calorie drinks, zero tab. salt

Fine Tuning of Ketogenic Diet

Once the KD is planned, there may be many questions the parents /caregivers might come across in the days to day routine. Therefore it should be kept in mind that just planning a diet does not end the task of the dietician's task. A lot of fine tuning may be required on individual basis and from time to time. Following are the general principles to be followed:

- Make only one change at a given time – either calories (usually 100/d) or ratio (usually 0.2-0.5)
- It might take 15-30 days to assess the effect
- Urine testing should be done regularly (3-4/days) and around the same time
- Ensuring charting to be done immediately
- The warning signs of excess ketosis should be explained to the parents.

Some of the problems which may arise at initiation of KD would revolve around the following factors which need readjustment:

- Caloric intake
- Keto ratio
- CHO ratio
- Use/misuse of free foods
- Recipe preparation
- Recipe presentation
- Fastidious eaters
- Fluid intake
- Processed food content
- Proper calculation of recipe
- Proper food values
- Intercurrent illness

Tube Feeding of KD

In children where tube feeding is required the following points need to be considered:

- Plan the feed based on the IBW and calories required. The recipes however would be different
- Same precautions of weighing ingredients are required as for other KD
- Oil/butter/ghee should not be premixed in the recipe but done so just before feeding
- The mixture should be brought to room temperature or made slightly warm before feeding
- After feeding the tube should be flushed with 10-15 ml of sterile water
- The vitamin supplements, if required should be added to the feeds
- Rest of the precautions required for any tube feeds, apply to feeding KD too.

Phase 4

After the child is initiated on the KD, it is essential to follow them up at regular intervals. The follow-up involves:

- Anthropometry: Weight and height at every visit
- Check ketone charts which are to be maintained by patients
- Recheck of ketone testing should be done at every visit
- Weighing scales to be evaluated for accuracy
- A variety of recipes to be planned and given to patients
- Problems of constipation/diarrhea or urine frequency to be addressed at every follow-up.

SIDE EFFECTS ON KD

As this diet is not as per the typical normal diet, certain side effects may occur in some patients, but all of them can be handled with the required adjustments. Side effects may be short-term or long-term as shown in Table 13.4.

Hypoglycemia: Generally seen in children who begin with fasting, especially in small babies. But currently fasting the child is not practiced. To manage the effect of hypoglycemia, blood sugars should be checked every 4 hours. In case the child is very sleepy, 30 ml of sugar free orange juice may be given. A carbohydrate wash out diet should be initiated rather than fasting before a KD.

Drowsiness: This can happen due to possible change in binding of certain anticonvulsants allowing higher concentration of these into the brain, causing lethargy or drowsiness in some children.

Dehydration: Fluid intake may be suboptimal, as in patients on KD, thirst is decreased and the child becomes more sedated. Therefore one should look for signs of dehydration. To manage this problem, plain water or soda with sugar free tablet with flavors like orange or sweet lime may be offered. Normal saline can also be given.

Nausea/Vomiting: When patients are fasted before starting on KD, followed by a high fat diet with ratio of 4:1, there may be excess of ketosis and acidosis which can cause vomiting. In some children long term used of foods like eggs, soya and excess of oil/ghee in the diet could cause vomiting. To manage the problem, fasting should be avoided and a lower keto ratio of fats to carbohydrates and proteins may be planned. Sucking of ice cubes before and after meals can reduce this problem. Plain soda with flavors (sugar free) before and after can help reduce the effect of vomiting. High ketosis causing vomiting may be managed by offering some orange juice (sugar free) before meals.

Constipation: This may occur due to a small volume of food which is very low in carbohydrates. A very low fiber and restricted fluids intake

Table 13.4: Side effects of ketogenic diet

Short-term early side effects	*Long-term side effects*
Hypoglycemia	Growth retrardation
Drowsiness	Anemia
Dehydration	Hypomagnesemia
Nausea/Vomiting	Zinc deficiency
Constipation	Osteopenia
Hyperuricemia	Hypercarotenemia

can also contribute to the problem. To manage this problem, fiber content may be increased by adding vegetables from Group A (Table 13.2A) in the diet. Laxatives which are sugar free can help alleviate the problem.

Crystalliuria: A high protein intake and restricted fluid intake can lead to formation of crystals in the urine. This can be corrected by increasing water or fluid intake and also reducing intake of purine rich foods like meats, pulses, beans, etc.

LONG-TERM SIDE EFFECTS

Growth retardation: Most children do lag behind the normal growth velocity due to restricted calories and proteins but once they are off the diet, they do catch-up with expected growth pattern.

Nutritional deficiency: Since the diet is not a normal diet, it tends to lack in some essential micronutrients, resulting in deficiency of some essential micronutrients, resulting in anemia, hypomagnesemia, selenium deficiency, zinc deficiency and osteopenia. It is therefore important to supplement these vitamins and minerals in their feeds.

Hyperlipidemia: The ketogenic diet being very high in fats, risk of hyperlipidemia cannot be ruled out. However, the adverse effects can be minimized by a judicious use of various fats and oils. The combination of fats is vital and also the ratio of various fats, rather than any one single fat, like groundnut oil and sunflower oil and ghee in the ratio of 2:1 in a 4 meal day (monounsaturated, polyunsaturated and saturated). Use of soybean oil is advocated due to its hypocholesterolemic effect. Good amount of fiber through fruits and vegetables can also help.

In general all complications of the KD are transient and can be managed easily with various conservative treatments. However, life threatening complications need to be monitored closely during follow-up.[13]

IMPORTANT FACTORS TO BE CONSIDERED ON KD

- Offer small/frequent meals (2-3 hourly)
- Use liberal fats /oils
- Use a combination of groundnut oil and sunflower oil in alternative recipes
- Use sugar free medications/tooth paste
- Supplement vitamins and minerals as required
- Soyapack once opened should be consumed within 24 hours
- In case of vomiting/decreased appetite, seek medical aid.

THE MEDIUM CHAIN TRIGLYCERIDES (MCT) KETO-DIET

This type of diet uses medium chain triglycerides (MCT) based fat in combination with the KD. The advantage of this is that the energy distribution is done as 30 percent from MCT, 30 percent from fat and 40 percent energy from combined natural foods which will provide proteins, carbohydrates and additional dietary fats. It could be 19 percent carbohydrates and 10 percent proteins and 11 percent other fats. Sources of MCT used are butter, ghee, mayonnaise olive oil, margarine, coconut oil and commercially available formulations (Simyl MCT). Success rate with use of MCT oil along with classified KD in some percentage to help achieve ketosis and also to increase the bulk of the diet. The advantage of MCT is that it allows more protein intake, includes more micronutrients and has fewer incidence of kidney stones or constipation. But there are certain disadvantages too of this diet as it was found to be very unpalatable thereby having lower compliance. Problems of abdominal cramps, severe diarrhea or nausea and vomiting may occur on this diet. Moreover it is more costly than the other diets.

Therefore it is recommended that MCT based KD be used in patients who:

- Are not on valporate or epival anticonvulsant as it may interfere with these drugs.
- Are not on gastric tube feeds.
- Have no problem of aspiration or diarrhea
- Are picky eaters
- Have large appetites
- Are older than 1 year.

Lastly MCT diet can be used in any ratio, based on individual tolerance and the need to improve seizure control.

DISCONTINUATION OF DIET

The diet may be weaned off or discontinued after 2-3 years on the diet, or after 6 months of seizure free period. This should be done gradually over a period of 2-3 months by lowering the keto ratio, till urinary ketosis is nil. Thereafter a free diet without any calorie restriction is allowed. But the rate of recurrence of seizures is expected in about 20 percent of the cases, over varying periods averaging 2 years. At certain centers this diet can be carried out for as long as possible or till the child is able to accept and tolerate it well. The policy may vary from one center to the other.

MODIFIED ATKINS DIET (MAD)

If the classical KD or the MCT based diets are too difficult to follow or too restrictive, the modified Atkins diet is an easier alternative to help control seizures. Although MAD was basically introduced for inducing weight loss, it has found a reasonable acceptability as an alternative to the classic KD. In this type of diet a consistent level of ketosis may not be achieved, but in older children, who may not comply with restrictions of a classical KD, MAD may be a more tolerable option.[14] It is typically a high fat, low carbohydrate diet, the advantages of which are:

- No fasting/hospitalization is required
- No calculations/weighing are required
- No limit to the amount and timings of eating
- Wider variety
- Does not require constant supervision of a doctor/dietician.

Table 13.5 highlights the major differences between the original and modified Atkins diet.

The list of foods allowed in MAD is as given in Table 13.6. There are certain points to be instructed to the care givers while preparing the MAD like:

- Chop vegetables in small pieces and deep fry chicken, eggs, fish, mutton, etc.
- Make cubes/toffees of butter. Freeze it and then grate or top it on recipes or use as garnishing
- Use ad lib oil/ghee for recipe preparations

The amount of carbohydrates permitted varies on the age of the child:

- 2-12 years old–allowed any 4 items/d, each containing 2.5 g CHO from the listed foods rich in CHO (vegetables, fruits, milk/milk products, nuts)
- >12 years old–allowed any 3 items/d each containing 5 g CHO
- The CHO exchange list to be used in MAD is as shown in Table 13.7.[11]

THE LOW GLYCEMIC INDEX TREATMENT (LGIT)

In the LGIT diet, stable blood glucose levels are attempted to be achieved, using a restricted diet. This is based on the hypothesis that blood glucose may be involved in achieving ketosis. This allows for greater freedom to use carbohydrates up to 40-60 g/d, which is more than in either the classic or the modified Atkins diet. The only restriction is the limit the carbohydrates of low glycemic index foods, i.e. up to 50 or less. Quite a few centers offer both the types of regimen – MAD and LGIT despite their limited trials, they have shown to be more accepted by adolescents.[15]

Table 13.5: Modified atkins diet versus classical ketogenic diet

Modified atkins diet	*Classic ketogenic diet*
High fat foods strongly encouraged amount of carbohydrates: 0-2 years – 5 g 2-12 years – 10 g > 12 years – 15 g Weight loss not the goal. Eat ad lib.	High fat foods are allowed. Carbohydrates 20 g/d for just 2 weeks. Weight loss is the main goal.

Table 13.6: Foods allowed in modified atkins diet

Carbohydrates	*Given in prescribed amounts*	*Vegetable/fruits, milk/milk products, nuts*
Fats/Proteins	Zero carb foods given freely (fats and protein foods)	Fats, oils, chicken, fish, eggs, soya products, homemade mayonnaise
Free	Zero calorie foods/Free foods	Sugar free jelly, zero calorie drinks, zero tab salt

Table 13.7: Carbohydrate exchange list in MAD

Fruits	*For children 2-12 yrs (any 4/d)*	*For adolescents and adults >12 yrs (any 3/d)*
Fruit A (apples, papaya, pear)	1 cup	2 cups
Fruit A (Orange, sweet lime)	3 pcs.	6 pcs.
Fruit A (Pomegranate)	3/4th cup	1.5 cups
Fruit A (Grapes)	6 pcs.	12 pcs.
Milk (Milk Products) Soya Milk (Natural Staeta)	2.5 cups	5 cups
Cow's Milk/Buffalo Milk	1 cup	2 cups
Paneer/Cheese	1-5 cubes	3 cubes
Cream	1 cup	2 cups
Nuts Almonds/Groundnuts	20 pcs.	40 pcs.
Walnuts	1 cup	2 cups
Coconut	1.5 tbsp	3 tbsp

Ref. J. Nathan (11)

REFERENCES

1. Ries LAGSM, Gurney JG, Tamira T, et al. Cancer incidence and survival among children and adolescents. United States SEER Program 1976-95, national Cancer Institute, SEER program NIH Pub Bethesda, MD, 1999;17-34.

2. Jensen C. New study suggests link between maternal diet and childhood leukemia risk. Science Daily. Aug 24, 2004.
3. Marilyn l Kwan, Gladys Block, Steve Selvin, Stacy Month and Patricia A Buffer. Food consumption by children and the risk of childhood acute leukemia. Am J Epidemiology, Vol 160, No. 11, pp 1098-1107.
4. www.cureepilepsy.org/psas/charlies_story.asp.
5. John WL, Puntis. Nutritional challenges in special conditions and diseases, Hemato Oncology In: Pediatric Nutrition in Practice, Ed. Koletzko B. Karger, 2008;244-47.
6. Oeffinger KC, Mertens AC, Sklar CA, et al. Obesity in adult survivors of childhood acute lympoblastic leukemia: A report from the Childhood Cancer Survivor Study. J Clin Oncol 2003; 21:1359-65.
7. Wharton BO, Bower BD, Schwartz RH, Eaton J and Aynsley Green A. The use of ketogenic diet in the treatment of epilepsy. In: Topics in Perinatal Medicine (ed) 1982;pp136-40.
8. Kossoff EH, Lau LC, Blackford R, Morrison PF, et al. When do seizures usually improve with ketogenic diet? Elipelsia 2008;49(20):329-33.
9. Wheless JW. History and origin of ketogenic diet. In: Stafstorm CE. Rho LM editors, Epiepsy and the ketogenic diet. Totowa: Humana Press:2004.
10. Livingston S, Charles C Thomas. Dietary treatment of epilepsy. In: Comprehensive management of epilepsy in infancy; Childhood and Adoescence. Springfield, Illinois: 1972;pp378-405.
11. J Nathan. Epilepsy and Keto Research Trust, Mumbai.
12, Gopalan C, Rama Sastri BV and Balasubramanian SC, Nutritive Value of Indian Foods. National Institute of Nutrition, ICMR, Hyderabad.
13. Zhou W, Mukherjee P, Kiebish MA, et al. The calorie restricted ketogenic diet, an alternative therapy for malignant brain cancer. Nutrition and Metabolism (London) 2007;4:5.
14. Kang HC, Lee HS, You SJ, Kangder C, Ko TS, Kim HD. Use of a modified Atkins diet in intractable epilepsy. Epilepsia 2007;48 (1):182-6.
15. Kossoff EH, Zupec-Kania BA, Amark PE, et al. Optimal clinical management of children receiving the ketogenic diet. Recommendations of the International Ketogenic Diet Study group. Epilepsia. 2008, Sep.23.

Chapter 14 Inborn Errors of Metabolism

PHENYLKETONURIA

Phenylketonuria (PKU) is a rare form of disorder, due to a recessive inherited metabolic disorder, first recognized in 1934 by Folling. In this condition, both parents are heterogeneous carriers and the risk of other children being involved is one in four.

The incidence varies from 1 in 10,000 in caucasians to 1 in 30,000 in newborns.[1]

The disorder involved a defect in the conversion of phenylalanine (Phe) to tyrosine, due to which there is an accumulation of phenylalanine in the blood and tissues resulting in excessive production of phenylketones. This results in children having retardation of developmental progress, severe mental retardation, hyperactivity, seizures, a light complexion and eczema. The urine has a mouse like odor.

The mechanism of conversion of phenylalanine to tyrosine in a normal and affected child has been depicted in Figure 14.1.

Due to low levels of hepatic phenylalanine hydroxylase phenylalanine cannot be converted to tyrosine. As a result there is accumulation of Phe in the blood, cerebrospinal fluid and the tissues. Due to this block in the normal metabolic pathway, accessory metabolic pathways develop, which convert Phe to phenylpyruvic acid and hydroxyphenyl acetic acid, which are then excreted in the urine. The subsequent accumalation of Phe and other metabolites in the serum, affects the utilization of other amino acids by the cells. This results in deprivation of essential and consequent retardation in the development of the brain.

However, prompt treatment of such children with diet restricted in Phe results in reversal of symptoms and leads to normal intellectual development. It is recommended not to delay dietary intervention beyond 2 days for good results.

PKU is known to be of two types:

- Classical
- Atypical

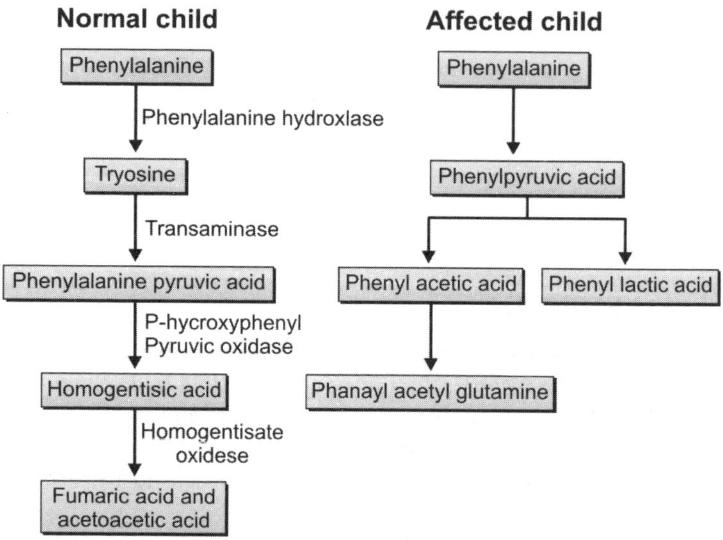

Fig. 14.1: Conversion of phenylalanine in a normal and affected child

In classical PKU, hepatic phenylalanine is low or absent and blood levels on a normal diet usually exceed 1200 μmol/l, but tyrosine levels are low or normal. The defect involves incomplete myelination of the central nervous sysyem. A classical case of PKU will not tolerate more than 400 mg of dietary phenylalanine per day. With this level of dietary Phe, blood Phe level of 480 μmol/l can be safely achieved.

In atypical PKU, the enzyme block is less complete than in classical condition. The blood Phe levels are usually less than 1200 μmol/l, although a high dietary protein intake or an acute catabolic episode may raise this figure. In general, these patients have a higher level of tolerance of dietary Phe, managing 2-3 times the quantity of natural protein tolerated by these with the classical form, when Phe levels are in safe range.[1]

DIAGNOSIS

Screening a child for PKU involves detection of raised Phe levels (upper limit of normal 240 μmol/l). In the cord blood these levels are generally normal, but begin to rise steadily after birth, following breastfeeding or even formula milk. In an unscreened child, the presenting symptoms could be seizures, albinism (excessively fair hair and skin) and a 'musty' odor to the baby's sweat, skin and urine. A tendency to hypopigmentation and eczema are also observed.

All patients with blood Phe levels greater than 240 μmol/l, should be investigated further. Infants on breastfeeds or otherwise should be evaluated for the protein content of their diet, as a high protein intake can artificially elevate Phe levels. The tests should be repeated after 2 weeks, to confirm the diagnosis but dietary modification can however be initiated earlier. Breastfeeding should be preferred to cow's milk as it has a lower Phe content.

DIETARY MANAGEMENT

Successful treatment of patients with PKU depends upon:

- Early diagnosis
- Restriction of Phe intake to maintain an acceptable range of serum levels
- A nutritionally adequate diet adjusted from time to time to meet the requirements for normal growth and development
- Continuing clinical and biochemical monitoring
- Education and counseling of parents.

Children diagnosed with PKU need closely monitored feeding to ensure that the protein levels of their diet does not exceed sharply, especially after weaning has been introduced. Table 14.1 gives the requirements in classical PKU patients.[2]

If breast milk is unavailable for some reason, whey based modified milk (commercially available) having the amino acid profile of human milk can be substituted. Breastfeeding infants have to be monitored for their Phe levels in blood and weight gain at weekly intervals. If the levels are between 180-480 μmol/l, there is no need to restrict breast milk and can be continued as for normal children. However, if Phe levels exceed >

Table 14.1: Requirements in classical PKU per Kg per day

Age (years)	*Energy (Kcals)*	*Protein (g)*	*Phenylalanine from Natural protein (mg)*
0-1	100-130	3.4	50-60
1-2	90-100	2.5-3.5	30-40
2-4	80-100	2-3	25-40
4-6	80-100	2-3	25
6-8	70-90	2-2.5	15-20
8-14	55-75	1-1.5	As tolerated
> 14	45	1	As tolerated

Ref. Hemalatha R. NIN, ICMR, Hydearbad, 1999[2]

200 μmol/l, breast milk is withheld for 2-3 days and a low phenylalanine food supplement (LPFS), protein substitute is initiated (Table 14.2). Some of the commercially available low Phe food supplements in the Western market are LPFS (low phenylalanine food supplement), PHFS (protein hydrolysate food supplement), PHFS plus minerals, under the brand names, Lofenalac, Aminogram, and Aminogram mineral respectively. LPFS is basically a casein based hydrolysate from which 95 percent of phenylalanine is removed. The major constituent of these supplements are unsaturated fat, carbohydrates, vitamins and minerals.

After around 5-6 months when weaning is initiated to begin with approximately 10 g of a rice based weaning food mixed with boiled water can be offered, followed by fruits, vegetables in small amounts. Gradually an exchange of 50 mg Phe food (Table 14.3), is introduced in combination with 3-4 feeds of LPFS per day, based on the blood Phe levels. The aim should be to maintain a ratio of 40-50 Kcals: 1 g protein.[2] The calories can be increased by use of oil, butter, etc. By 6 months the protein requirement is increased, therefore protein hydrolysate food supplement (PHFS) is fed, gradually increasing the quantity from 1 tsp/d to

Table 14.2: Breastfeeding regime for infants with PKU

Blood Phenylalanine 15 percent Sol	*LPFS*	*Breastfeeds μmol/l*
> 2000	150-200 ml/Kg/d	Nil for 3 days
1200-2000	150-200 ml/Kg/d	Nil for 2 days
After 2 days, 45 ml-5 feeds		
< 1200	30 ml-5 feeds	On demand
480-900	15 ml-5 feeds	On demand

Ref. Hemalatha R. NIN, ICMR, Hyderabad, 1999[2]

Table 14.3: Amount of natural foods providing 50 mg of phenylalanine (weighed after cooking)

Food item	*Quantity*
Milk	50 ml
Potatoes (boiled)	75 g
Potatoes (chips)	30 mg
Pear (fresh)	20 mg
Cornflakes	15 mg
Wheatflakes	10 mg
Rice (boiled)	54 mg
Porridge (with water)	65 mg
Tomato sauc	50 mg
Wheat (roasted)	25 mg

Ref. Hemalatha R. NIN, ICMR, Hyderabad, 1999[2]

1 tsp 3 times a day, then eventually full dose of 3g PHFS per Kg/d along with 8g PHFS mineral supplements as given in Table 14.4. Breastfeeds and LPHS are proportionately reduced and finally omitted. Gradually solids are increased as per the requirement for age and blood levels of Phe. The daily intake of cow's milk or pasteurized fresh milk is divided and exchanged with LPFS. The total volume of feeds should not exceed 150-200 ml/kg/d.[2]

It has also been stressed that a balance must be maintained between the amount of low Phe formula and the amount of natural foods that are fed. An inadequate amount of Phe can lead to signs of deficiency which include anorexia, vomiting, listlessness, inconsistent growth or failure to gain weight, pallor and skin rash.[3] The low Phe formula like Lofenac supplies most of the energy, proteins and other nutrients and if inadequate amounts are fed, the amino acids and other nutrient requirements of the child will not be met. On the other hand, if inadequate amounts of natural foods are given, the Phe intake will be too low to meet the requirements. Although Phe intake is restricted, it must be remembered that this is one of the essential amino acids.

Low Phenylalanine Diet for 1-4-year-old Children

By 1 year of age the child should be consuming 5-6 times per day comprising 3 main meals and 2-3 snacks per day as shown in Table 14.4. Unfortunately, the low Phenylalanine supplements are yet not available in India; therefore in the absence of these, most children show deterioration of symptoms, in spite of early diagnosis.

ATYPICAL PHENYLKETONURIA

Children diagnosed with atypical PKU, if at all require treatment, need to follow more or less the same principles as for 'classical phenylketonuria, but the protein can be more liberal with a wider selection of foods and less of low Phe protein substitutes prescribed. However, these children need to be reassessed-up to 1 year of age to consider the feasibility of allowing them a near normal diet.

According to observations, children with atypical symptoms, PKU treated for varying periods of time, with blood levels, 600 µmol/l generally continue to be normal even after withdrawal of low Phe diets.[1] Nevertheless, parents should be apprised of the risks of maternal PKU, in case of female patients.

The National Society for PKU (UK) has formulated a list of foods allowed and restricted for patients with PKU which include detailed

Table 14.4: Low phenylalanine diets for children (1-4 years)

Age	*1 month*	*8 months*	*2 years*	*4 years*
Weight (Kg)	3.63	8.2	11.8	16.3
Diet Advised				
Phenylalanine (mg)	160-176	324-360	416-468	360-576
Protein (g)	14-16	27	32	40
Calories (Kcals)	440	810	1300	1700
LPFS measures (15g)	10	18	19	23
Water (to make-up volume to)	24 oz	32 oz	24 oz	24 oz
Milk	1-1/2 oz	1oz	-	-
Vegetables	-	2	4	4
Fruits	-	1	4	4
Rice/wheat exchange	-	3	5	5
Fat exchange	-	-	As desired	As desired
Free foods, US Dept				
Nutritive Value				
Phenylalanine (mg)	172	325	417	447
Protein (g)	16.8	30.4	33.1	40.4
Calories	540	944	1302	1724

Ref. Acosta PB: Nutritional aspects of Phenylketonuria. In: The clinical team looks at Phenylketonuria. Children's Bureau, US. Dep't of Health, Education and Welfare, Washington DC, p52.

dietary information for treatment of PKU.[4] They have formulated a traffic light system based on the colors of various foods to be included or excluded. These are:

Red........ Stop! – Do not eat at all
Amber... Go cautiously–Foods to be eaten in moderate amounts
Green .... Go! – These foods may be eaten in normal amounts
The foods included under the various lights are:

Red List

Foods high in Phe to avoid–meats, fish, eggs, cheese, nuts, breadflour, cakes, biscuits, soya based foods, aspartame (artificial sweetener found in most fizz drinks, cokes, squashes, chewing gums and some drugs).

Amber List

Foods containing some Phe to be taken with caution. Basic list of some exchanges of food to be followed should be measured accurately (Table 14.4).

Green List

Fruits: Apple, banana (1 small), dates, apricots, fresh and dried, blackberries, cherries, currants, figs, grapes, guavas, lemon, kiwi, mangoes, melon (water, musk), oranges, peaches, pineapple, plums, raisins, raspberries, strawberries.

Vegetables: Beans, beetroot, cabbage, cauliflower, carrots, celery, cucumber, ladyfingers, lettuce, mushrooms, mustard, onions, peppers (red, yellow, green), pumpkin, radish, sweet potato, tomato, turnip.

Cereals: Cornflour, arrowroot, custard powder, sago, tapioca.

Fats: Butter, vegetable oils, margarine (but not the one containing buttermilk).

Miscellaneous: Sugar-white, brown, castor, jam, honey, marmalade, baking powder, soda bicarbonate, cream of tartar, vegetarian jellies without gelatin.

Beverages: Soda water, mineral water, lemonade, squashes, tea, coffee, pine fruit, juices, coke (without aspartame).

GALACTOSEMIA

Galactosemia is another inborn error of metabolism and as the name suggests involves accumulation of galactose in the blood, which otherwise in the normal state gets converted to glucose in the liver. The defect involves:

- Absence of an enzyme, galactose-1-phosphate uridyl transferase, which is needed in the liver for the conversion.
- Deficiency of galactokinase which catalyses the formation of galactose-1-phosphate from galactose.

Galactose is a derivative of glucose and lactose and is derived from the hydrolysis of lactose in the intestine. Most dietary galactose is derived from lactose, the disaccharide of milk that is hydrolysed to galactose and glucose by the action of intestinal lactase, which is usually normal in these patients. Analysis of the RBC shows little or no transferase in those who have this disorder and half the normal levels in those who are carriers. This enzyme defect is inherited as an autosomal recessive trait and mothers of galactosemic infants have a diminished ability to metabolize galactose. Such mothers, if they consume excess amounts of milk during pregnancy, the possibilities of damage to the fetus exist, as galactose may pass the placenta.[5]

CLINICAL PRESENTATION

Children are normal at birth, but after a few days of birth with introduction of milk (breast or formula) symptoms like vomiting, anorexia, occasional diarrhea, drowsiness, jaundice, puffiness of face, edema of the lower extremities and weight loss begin to appear. Poor sucking is observed within 48 hours of birth. Without treatment the outcome is generally fatal, but if the child does survive, chances of developing mental retardation, cirrhosis of liver and cataract are quite high. However, early diagnosis and prompt dietary intervention can lead to excellent immediate results and a favorable long-term prognosis. Diagnosis is confirmed by elevated levels of galactose-1-phosphatase in erythrocytes, which is thought to be a toxic metabolite, proteinuria, aminoaciduria and raised serum galactose and urinary galactose with depressed blood glucose levels. Cataracts may be present at birth or develop subsequently and may remain irreversible despite treatment.

DIETARY MANAGEMENT

Dietary exclusion of galactose and lactose sources is the only intervention to prevent clinical symptoms and ensure normal growth and development. Milk especially human milk is very high in galactose and therefore breastfed infants manifest symptoms very early. A nutritionally adequate diet free of all milk sources needs to be incorporated. Substitution of non milk formula leads to rapid improvement. All symptoms except mental retardation disappear. There are controversial opinions regarding use of soya milk as a substitute. Some authors have used it successfully while others opine that stachyose, a terasaccharide in soyabeans, is hydrolysed to galactose. Rice based formulae or other commercially available milk free baby foods need to be fed till such time the child is old enough to accept other cereal-pulse based diets. These formulae need to be supplemented with calcium, iron and vitamins. Care should be taken to avoid all milk based foods like, ice cream, bread, biscuits, puddings, chocolates, butter, margarine, toffees, etc.

By the time the child is 6-8 months old, a greater variety of foods can be available, e.g. rice, dal, khichdi, suji halwa or upma, dalia, etc. Introduction of eggs can be delayed till about 10-12 months and then given 2-4 times per week. A sample menu of a day's diet for toddlers and young children is presented in Table 14.5. Older children can gradually be permitted foods containing traces of lactose, but visible milk in the form of ice cream, custard, porridge, etc. should still be best avoided. Care should be taken to scrutinize all labels of all commercial products

Table 14.5: Galactose free diet for toddlers and young children sample menu

Breakfast	Cereal (suji halwa/choori, parantha/idli/dosa Egg—optional
Mid morning	Fruit/poha/besan pura/cheela
Lunch	Rice/chapati Dal Vegetable Tofu (soya based) Salad
Evening	Juice Idli/dosa/upma/suji halwa/veg. cutlet
Dinner	Khichdi/rice/chapatti Dal/chicken/fish Potato fingers Dessert (milk free)

Note: Use only refined vegetable oil/coconut oil

used or, when outdoor on social gatherings, the contents of the dishes included should always be verified.

DURATION OF DIETARY TREATMENT

In the initial years, dietary treatment is very strict, but as the child grows older, the diet may be relaxed to an extent to allow minimal lactose in their diets. The enzyme defect persists for life and hence children with galactosemia growing to adolescence and adulthood should always be wary of the selection of foods in their diet. In females, especially during pregnancy, restriction of lactose containing foods is advisable to avoid consequences in the newborn.

It is not very difficult to adhere to a lactose free diet for adolescents and adults as by then they have a greater variety of foods to choose from and milk and milk products is one small portion of any adult diet. With the exception of milk and milk products as a direct source, rest all other food groups can be incorporated in the menu of such patients as listed in Table 14.6.

As with PKU, dietary counseling is of great importance. Close rapport with parents and the children along with regular follow-up visits, helps in successful implementation of dietary compliance. Regular blood galactose estimates help to establish that normal limits are not exceeded.

FRUCTOSEMIA

Fructosemia is an inborn error manifesting somewhat like galactosemia. In this disorder, introduction of fructose in the diet of the infant before

Table 14.6: List of foods to be included and excluded in galactosemia

Foods	*Included*	*Excluded*
Milk group	Soya milk/curd, tofu (soya paneer)	All milk and milk products including breast milk, curd
Cereals/pulses	All cereals/pulses	
Fats/oils	Vegetable oils, butter, cream, ghee margarine without milk margarine with milk	
Fruits/vegetables	Fresh fruits/vegetables, peas, canned vegetables	
Meat group	Muscle meat, egg, fish, poultry, liver	
Miscellanous	All cold drinks, juices, dry fruits, all sweets from khoya, milk, sweets without, milk, khoya paneer, cheese, ice cream, besan products, sugar, custard, baby food supplements with whey/ casein, Jaggery	

6 months of age, results in anorexia, vomiting, failure to thrive, hypoglycemia, seizures and dysfunction of liver and kidneys.[6] Older children generally remain asymptomatic or may manifest with spontaneous hypoglycemia, which is believed to be caused by reduced glycogenolysis and gluconeogenesis.

The disorder involves four enzymes in fructose metabolism-hexokinase, fructokinase, fructaldose and fructose-1, 6-diphosphatase. Deficiency of the latter three has been described, but fructokinase deficiency is a benign error of metabolism and does not warrant any dietary restriction.

Hereditary fructose intolerance (HFI): This is due to the deficiency of primary fructaldolase deficiency in which fructose-1-phosphate accumulates. Clinical symptoms appear on first exposure to fructose (or sucrose) generally after weaning has been initiated with foods like fruit or sweetened cereals. Mostly such patients develop a strong aversion to sweet taste, therefore unintentional fructose intake is rare.

The striking feature of HFI, are fructosemia, fructosuria and hypoglycemia with symptoms of shock on ingestion of fructose. Once diagnosed, treatment should be initiated immediately continued for life by excluding fructose, sucrose and sorbitol from the diet. Elimination of fructose from the diet brings about immediate remission of symptoms except for hepatomegaly which may take greater time to resolve[7]

Table 14.7: List of foods included and excluded in HFI

Foods included	*Foods excluded*
Milk, cheese, cream, butter, curd	Sweetened condensed milk, infant feed. Eggs, fish chicken containing sucrose, commercial ice cream sweetened milk shakes
Rice, wheat flour, barley, oats, suji, dalia, cream,	Flavoured milk
Tapioca, bread only 2-3 slices/day	Flavoured and fruit yogurt
Cakes, biscuits made from glucose, soya and soya flour	Baby cereals, breakfast cereals, dextrins sweetened
Glucose and glucose drinks, starch, maltose	Custard, pudding mixes
Saccharine, aspartame	Cakes, biscuits, pastries,
Tea, coffee, cocoa (unsweetened) fruit sugar, invert sugar, honey syrup	All fruits/juices, tomato, jam, Caramel, marmalades
Vegetables-all except root vegetables, beans, peas, sweet corn, carrots, sorbitol/fructose, butter, ghee	
Salt, pepper, spices, vinegar, nuts, permitted ingredients paste/puree	Sorbitol, sweetening agents containing sucrose
	Jelly, tooth paste with sucrose or foods of doubtful content

Minimal inclusion of fructose in the diet can cause chronic symptoms of failure to thrive, hypoglycemia and liver diseases. A list of foods to be included and excluded in HFI is listed in Table 14.7.

Fructose-1-diphosphatase deficiency: In this deficiency symptoms include hypoglycemia, hyperventilation, hepatomegaly, failure to thrive, vomiting and seizures. Presence of lactic acidosis puts the infants at great risk. Unlike In HFI, these patients do not have aversion to sweet foods. In these children, glycogen is not metabolized normally and cannot be used to maintain glucose homeostasis. Unlike in HFI, where fasting improves symptoms, in patients with fructose-1-diphosphatase deficiency, fasting can cause hypoglycemia, therefore care needs to be taken avoid prolonged fasting in such patients. Frequent carbohydrate intake is very essential to maintain normoglycemia even when the child is well. A late night snack of starch based carbohydrate (sucrose and fructose free) is advisable. The total dietary carbohydrate should be high, approximately $\geq$ 65 percent of dietary energy and fat intake slightly restricted. Early diagnosis and prompt treatment can prevent irreversible damage.

FRUCTOSE FREE DIET

Fruits are the main source of fructose as also invert sugars which are a component of sucrose; therefore these must be excluded (including cane, beet or brown sugar, icing sugar and syrup, honey, all fruits, root vegetables, pulses and tomatoes). Some of the tooth pastes also contain some fructose and sucrose from natural fruits and need to be avoided. Other fructose or sucrose containing foods include diabetic sweets which use sorbitol, chocolates and squashes. All medicines in liquid form may contain sucrose or sorbitol and must be replaced by alternatives. A list of foods allowed and restricted is presented in Table 14.7.

MAPLE SYRUP DISEASE (MSUD)

This disease also termed as branched chain ketoaciduria relates to biochemical defect and is an autosomal recessive disease. The missing factor is the enzyme oxidative decarboxylase in white blood corpuscles (WBC). As such the carboxyl group cannot be removed resulting in accumulation of amino acids and ketoacids in the urine. This gives the typical odor of maple syrup to the urine and hence the name. At birth the child appears normal but becomes symptomatic within first few days of life. They experience sucking problems; respiration is irregular with intermittent periods of rigidity and flaccidity. Seizures of the grand mal type are present, and if the child survives, may manifest with mental disorders. Hyperglycemia is frequently encountered in these children and due to increased tissue catabolism following infection, there is further rise in the accumalation of the offending metabolites in the circulation.

Dietary Management

Management comprises a diet restricted in the branch chain amino acids, which is only in commercial formulation. However, a formula suited specifically for such needs is not yet available in India. Small amounts of milk may be continued in view of the requirements for growth and development. The guidelines for management of PKU can be adapted for this disorder. Most fruits and vegetables are permitted having more or less 50 mg leucine per 100 g. These are apples, pineapple, raisins, banana (in limited amount), carrots, beans, cabbage, onion, pumpkin, tomato, beetroot and turnips.

HOMOCYSTINURIA

This also is an autosomal recessive disorder and in which the enzyme cystathionine synthetase is lacking. The enzyme is present in the liver and brain and is necessary for conversion of homocysteine to cystathione, an intermediate product formed in the metabolism of methionine. The manifestations are mental disorder along with cataract and dissolution of muscles of the pelvic girdle, thrombosis and pulmonary embolism are commonly seen in these patients.

Dietary Modifications

The diet should be modified for low methionine, high cystine content. Gelatin is a good source of protein being low in methionine. It is supplemented with synthetic amino acids like leucine, isoleucine, tryptophan and valine.

WILSON'S DISEASE

Wilson's disease is a hereditary autosomal recessive disorder which involves degeneration of the hepatic cells. The defect involves very low serum levels of ceruloplasmin, a copper containing protein of the blood. This is due to the increased absorption of copper from the GI tract and an increased deposit of copper in the brain, liver and kidney.

Age of presentation is generally between 4-5 years or in some can be as late as the first decade of life also. The clinical manifestations in these patients are ascites, jaundice, live enlargement and neurological involvement. The child might show a blank dazed look with the presence of tremors, seizures and dementia. A typical diagnostic feature is the presence of Kayser-Fleischer (KF) ring in the eye (a greenish brown discoloration).

Dietary Modifications

Management in such children involves dietary modifications which involves avoiding high copper food sources. Chelating agents are used to chelate or break away the copper of the diet, thus minimizing the absorption from the GIT. The aim should be to maintain a level of 1 mg copper or less in the diet. The normal range generally is about 2-3 mg.

Most foods have some amounts of copper present, but high sources are organ meats, shellfish, mushrooms, legumes, whole grain cereals, nuts, chocolates and colas. All commercial and tinned foods should be restricted. A significant source of copper can be leached out from copper vessels used for boiling milk in a majority of Indian households, especially if they are not adequately tinned. Therefore mothers should be warned against using copper vessels for cooking or storing milk or any other food item to be consumed by the child.

Table 14.8: Foods restricted and allowed in Wilson's disease

Foods restricted (High copper-0.8-1mg percent)	*Foods allowed (Low copper-0.01-0.6 mg percent)*
All dry fruits, nuts (coconut, peanuts)	All cereals-rice, wheat, maize
All seeds-til, mustard, saffola oil	All leafy vegetables, green peas
All organ meats-liver, kidney	All fruits
Chocolates, toffees, colas	All roots, tubers and other vegetables
Black pepper, gram whole, Bengal gram	Pulses-whole moong dal, arhar
White and kabuli gram, lentil, dry peas	Fish
rajma, moth dal	Milk and milk products
Mushrooms	Fats and sugars

Treatment depends upon low copper diet (1.0-1.8 mg/24 hours), preventing copper absorption, mobilizing these deposits and promoting their excretion. Potassium sulfide, 20 mg, three times a day with meals, prevents copper absorption.[8] Patients with Wilson's disease may develop anemia, therefore iron supplements need to be given also. Zinc given orally increases fecal copper excretion.[9] Table 14.8 presents a picture of the foods to be avoided and allowed in patients with Wilson's disease.

REFERENCES

1. Dorothy EM Francis. Phenylketonuria In: Diets for Sick Children, 4th ed. Blackwell Scientific Publications 1987;224-62.
2. Hemalatha R. Diet Therpay in classical Phenylketonuria, Nutrition, National Institute of Nutrition, ICMR, Hyderabad, April 1999.
3. Sutherland BS, et al. Growth and nutrition in treated phenylketonuric patients. JAMA 1970;211:270-6.
4. National Society for Phenylketonuria (UK), London N14 4ZF, Compant No: 1256124, Charity No: 273670.
5. Hansen RG. Hereditary Galactosemia. JAMA 1969;208:2077-82.
6. Levin B, et al. Fructosemia. Observations on seven cases. Am J Med. 1968;45:826-38.
7. Burman D, Holten JB, Pennock CA. Baerlocher K, Gitzelmann R, Steinmann B. In: Inherited Disorders of carbohydrate metabolism. Eds. 1980;pp 163-90. Lancaster. MTP press Ltd.
8. FP Antia. Copper In: Clinical Dietetics and Nutrition, 3rd ed, Oxford University Press Bombay 1993;pp 125-7.
9. Brewer GJ, Hills GM, Prasad AS, Cossack ZT, et al. Oral zinc therapy for Wilson's disease. Ann Intern Med 1983;99:314-20.

Chapter 15 Diet in Liver Diseases

The liver is the largest and most complex organs of the body, involved in multiple functions of nutrient absorption and metabolism like proteins, carbohydrates and lipids besides vitamins and minerals. It is also involved in the detoxification of bacterial decomposition products, mineral poisons and certain drugs and dyes. Any insult on the liver can have direct bearing on the nutritional status of an individual, more so on the child.

When the liver is affected by any infection, it results in the inflammation of the hepatic cells, causing hepatitis. In children, hepatitis is generally infective, caused mainly by infective agents from food and water. Other causes of hepatitis could be metabolic or nutritional, or biliary obstruction. The pathologic changes involved in the liver parenchymal cells are similar regardless of the etiology of the disease.[1]

HEPATITIS

Etiology

Hepatitis in children is generally due to infections, characterized by inflammatory and degenerative changes in the liver. The infective type is mostly due to viral cause, or it may be drug induced due to A, B, C, D, E or any of the numerous types identified. Amongst them hepatitis A is the most commonly identified, which is transmitted through the fecal oral route. Epidemics are generally seen from time-to-time either by fecal contamination of water or a breakdown in the sanitation system. Serum hepatitis is transmitted only through the parenetral route in blood products containing the specific virus or through faulty sterilization of needles. Drug induced hepatitis may be due to hypersensitivity to certain drugs like sulfa or penicillin or due to a direct toxic affect on the liver by agents like carbon tetrachloride or certain herbal drugs containing alkaloids.

Symptoms

Children with hepatitis A may have symptoms varying from very mild in younger ones to more severe forms in older children. Since, the average incubation period could be for about 1 month before the onset of the symptoms, it may appear that the onset has been rather sudden. These include:

- Fatigue
- Vomiting and nausea
- Loss of appetite
- Low grade fever
- High colored urine with stools appearing very pale, giving a clay colored appearance
- Muscle pain
- Itching
- Yellow coloration of the skin and the conjunctiva.

Management

As of now no specific treatment exists for hepatitis A. The main focus is on adequate rest and nutrition and avoids any permanent liver damage. Complete recovery may take a few months.

Dietary modifications: The main objective of dietary treatment is to aid regeneration of the liver tissue and avoid further complications.

Calories: The energy requirement of a child with hepatitis is almost same as that for a normal healthy child. Though the child may be very anorexic or nauseated, it is advisable that small frequent feedings be encouraged to meet the nutritional goal. This could be in the form of any type of diet which the child may prefer. It may be kept in mind that there should be no restrictions on the type of food the child may like. Usually parents tend to impose a lot of restrictions on the type of diet or foods the child should be having. The trend is mostly on highly sweetened foods, e.g. cane sugar juice or radish extract. These may actually cause the child to be more nauseated and deter him from eating at all.

The aim should be to maintain the normal weight of the child and also encourage weight gain if possible in the younger ones. Extremely over weight and obese children with viral hepatitis can add further complications to the liver, such as fatty deposits in the liver and accompanying liver inflammation called nonalcoholic steatohepatitis. An adequate amount of complex carbohydrates, e.g. rice, wholemeal breads, potatoes, sago and wholegrain cereals, can provide calories and help maintain weight for those children who are unable to maintain body mass. Adequate rest and moderate activity can also help.

Proteins: Adequate protein intake is important to maintain muscle mass and to regenerate the liver cells. The requirement for such children is as for any other normal child. There is no need for extra proteins nor should it be inadequate which can hinder the regenerative process of the liver.

***Carbohydrates*:** As mentioned earlier, the calorie requirement can be met only if there are adequate complex carbohydrate in the diets of such children. In contrast to the practice of loading children with hepatitis with too much of fruit juices, or cane sugar juice, a mixed carbohydrate diet is more acceptable and better tolerated by such children. This could be in the form of any of the day-to-day commonly consumed foods, which include sugars and fats. Since, in most of these children their appetite is severely compromised, care should be taken not to pressurize the child to eat. On the contrary, they should be given freedom to choose from any of the foods of their choice, be it in the form of sweets, savoury, cakes, pastries or pasta, noodles or pizzas topped with vegetables. The only care to be taken is to ensure the hygiene and safety of the source of the foods to avoid further complications of infections.

Fats: There is no restriction on the amount of fats to be allowed to a child with viral hepatitis. There is a general belief that fats should be restricted in patients suffering from viral hepatitis and hence offered boiled vegetables and other preparations. On the contrary, the appetite of the child is already compromises and in such a condition offering of boiled unpalatable food would only cause more aversion to food. This is the main reason why children affected by viral hepatitis after complete recovery, generally appear very undernourished, weak and fail to gain weight as per the desired velocity. The recommendations are normal fats (not too much or too little), as is advised for any normal child, i.e. 25 percent of the total calories. Moreover, incorporating small helpings of butter or cream in the preparations served can help increase the density of the food without adding to the bulk of their diet.

Vitamins and minerals: The requirement of all vitamins and minerals remain unchanged as for a normal healthy child. But due to the poor intake by the child, usually certain vitamins and minerals may be compromised and not being met. Care should be taken to avoid iron supplements to such children as it is known to reduce the response rate in patients with hepatitis C virus. It may also cause increased liver enzymes which indicate liver cell damage.[2]

Supplements/alternative medicine: The liver is responsible for the metabolism of medications and drugs. There are certain drugs and medicines, especially the herbal variety which can be toxic to the liver. Therefore, parents of children with viral hepatitis must refrain from giving any kind of supplements of herbal origin or any such medicines available over the counter, without discussing with their physician.

Alcohol: Intake of alcohol can precipitate liver toxicity and cause further damage to the liver cells. As children with chronic viral hepatitis approach adolescence, they need to be counseled regarding the dangers of alcohol to their health. The danger is magnified for the affected adolescent or teenager.

It should be kept in mind that viral hepatitis in children can be just like any other infective disease, but the management is quite simple and may not involve too many medications. It is more or less self-limiting in duration and may take about 1-2 months for the child to recover completely. A small number of children with hepatitis A may have relapses over 6-9 months period. The mainstays of management involve rest, a healthy balanced unrestricted diet as per the likings of the child and avoid any outdoor or uncooked food likely to be from doubtful source. Fruit juice extracted at home and fruits bought whole, can take care of the vitamins, besides providing carbohydrates and fiber.

Foods that can be offered to a child with viral hepatitis are as follows:

Cereals: Any breakfast cereal like bread, cornflakes, dalia, poha, suji or chapatti/parantha (if the chid demends). Noodles, past and, macaroni may be included for variety.

Pulses: All dals, washed/whole/dehusked in the form of dals with meals, gram flour in the for of any snacks or sprouts or as per the liking of the child.

Vegetables: All seasonal vegetables including green leafy vegetables can be offered in the form of vegetable cutlets or attractive sandwiches or vegetable soups. Potatoes can be incorporated in a number of dishes in a variety of forms-baked, boiled or mashed.

Fruits: Fruits as a whole are preferable. Fruit juice also can be offered to give a change in the palate. Fruit salad with cream can be an attractive option.

Milk/Milk products: Normal dairy milk used at home is suitable. It can be give as milk shakes, puddings or porridge, curd, cottage cheese in various forms depending upon the child's preference.

Nonvegetarian foods: Eggs, fish and chicken can be offered in any form incorporated with meals or as snacks. Red meat and pork should however be avoided.

Fats: All normal fats used in cooking at home may be used in normal amounts. Cream/butter too may be incorporated in various dishes depending upon the recipe and the child's preference.

Sugars: Simple sugars can be used in normal amounts as per the child's likings or habit. Sweet preparations in any form can add variety in the menu.

Sodium: In infective hepatitis in the absence of ascites, no restriction of sodium is advocated, therefore normal salt as per liking can be used.

CIRRHOSIS OF LIVER

Cirrhosis of the liver in children is diagnosed as a waxing and waning course of acute hepatitis. In children cirrhosis is known to occur in those with chronic hepatitis leading to liver cell damage gradually, over a period of more than 8 weeks. It is characterized by jaundice, ascites, hepatomegaly and altered liver function tests. In a few children the condition may lead to fulminant hepatic failure which is characterized by massive necrosis of the liver cells and severe impairment of liver function tests. The child may present with encephalopathy and has a high mortality and morbidity rate.[3]

Nutrition plays an important role in determining the outcome of the disease. The goals of nutritional management of cirrhosis in children are:

- Prevention and treatment of malnutrition by improving growth and development
- Reducing risk of hypoglycemia, infection and encephalopathy
- Avoid potential toxins in specific disorders
- Optimize nutritional status prior to transplant if indicated.

Energy: The energy level of a child with cirrhosis should be as high as 130 percent of the RDA. If this goal is difficult to achieve, nasogastric feeding may be resorted to.

Proteins: In the presence of hepatic encephalopathy, proteins are reduced in the diet, to not more than 1 g/Kg body weight, as drastic restriction can affect the growth and maintenance of the nitrogen (N) balance. Restriction of proteins has been attributed to poor growth and malnutrition. The proteins however, should be of high biological value which can be casein based preferably. Vegetable protein source is always advised as these are better tolerated than the animal proteins which are low in branched chain amino acids (BCCA). Moreover, consumption of vegetable proteins can alter the bowel flora with a beneficial effect.

At the same time excess of dietary protein also should be avoided as it can precipitate encephalopathy. A balanced vegetarian diet therefore is the mainstay of dietary management of cirrhosis in children, containing the required amounts of carbohydrates, fats, proteins and calories as per their age.

However, in the absence of encephalopathy, a high protein (casein based), of 2-3 g/Kg/d, should be emphasized, which is required for the speedy regeneration of the hepatocytes. This will also help in easing the associated edema and ascites due to hypoproteinemia. High protein supplements with BCCA may prove beneficial at this stage to augment the calorie and protein intake of the child. With BCCA enriched formulae, normal to high protein intakes do not cause encephalopathy. Vegetable proteins are high in BCCA, while animal proteins are not.[4] Studies have shown that enteral feeding with 4 g/kg/d of protein and 140 percent of the RDA of caloric intake in children with chronic liver disease led to improvement of nutritional status without hyperammonuria or any adverse affects.[5]

Carbohydrates: As these children are unable to store glycogen adequately, it is advisable they be fed a high carbohydrate diet which can be spread evenly over the day as it can delay the carbohydrate absorption resulting in its sustained release. Night time feeding of carbohydrates in the form of glucose polymer or uncooked starch can help maintain the glycogen stores and avoid the child going into hypoglycemia.

Fats: The fat content of the diet during the cirrhotic phase should not be reduced as it can make thc food unpalatable for the already anorexic child. Medium chain triglycerides can be given in emulsified form. The concept of low fat is no longer advisable as it was observed that low fat diets, besides reducing the palatability, also lowers the energy density of the diet. Children and adults are known to tolerate fats fairly well, therefore a low fat diet would only compromise the energy intake of the child. Inadequate energy will further affect the protein utilization due to the protein sparing affect. Coconut oil is a good example of MCT fats. Other sources are palm kernel oil and commercial MCT solution available as Simyl MCT. These are rapidly broken down in the small intestine and directly absorbed into the portal circulation being relatively more water soluble. But, since MCT oils are low in essential fatty acids, supplementation of these is required. Using a portion of fat as long chain triglycerides (LCT) in the form of safflower or corn oil can compensate for the deficiency. This is especially applicable to the child with cholestasis. This is applicable in a child with chronic cholestasis also which may be due to primary or secondary biliary cirrhosis, sclerosing cholangitis and biliary atresia.

Fat soluble vitamin supplements like vitamins A, D, E and K also need to be given to such children as they are known to malabsorb these vitamins.

Infants on breastfeeds should be allowed to continue as long as possible or up to a maximum of 2 years along with oral solid feeds.

Sodium: Children with cirrhosis, usually present with ascites too due to fluid retention. The pathogenesis involved may be either low plasma albumin due to defective synthesis, low osmotic pressure of plasma, hepatic venous outflow obstruction, and increased lymph exudation from the liver surface, increased renin aldosterone and low urinary excretion of sodium. All these factors lead to retention of salt and water.[3]

The principles of nutritional therapy in a child with cirrhosis may be summed up as follows.[6]

- Energy .... 125 percent of RDA (MCT/Glucose polymer)
- EFA..................... supplementation—corn/safflower oil
- Proteins.............. 2-3 g/Kg/d. BCC enriched diet-Albumin infusions
- Vitamin A .... 3000-10,000 IU/d orally.
- Vitamin D.......... 400-4000 IU/d orally.
- Vitamin E .... 50-400 IU/d orally.
- Vitamin K.......... 5 mg every 1-2 weeks IM.
- Calcium .... supplements as required.
- Phosphorus .... supplements as required
- Magnesium........ supplements as required.
- Zinc .... 1 mg/Kg/d
- Iron .... 3-5 mg/Kg/d
- Selenium............ 1-2 μ/Kg/d

INDIAN CHILDHOOD CIRRHOSIS (ICC)

Indian childhood cirrhosis as the name suggests, is one of the types of cirrhosis identified among Indian children where large amounts of copper deposition was reported. However, currently a very small proportion of children are encountered, probably due to the preventive measures adopted by households regarding use of copper/brass vessels for boiling milk for infants.

The disease was identified by Bernard Portman in 1978, in a series of children form Pune, who had liver disorders and was seeking evidence for hepatitis B infection. The confirmatory diagnosis was made by orcein staining which detects copper loading.[7]

Liver copper concentrations of 787-6654 μ/g dry weight were found in a series of children with ICC from Pune.[8]

It was postulated that hepatic copper retention may occur secondary to holestasis, but this was rejected since cholestasis was not a marked clinical feature and jaundice was a late clinical feature.

Etiology/Source

Studies from Pune group of workers discovered on reviewing the background of all the patients suffering from ICC, that all of them belonged to rural communities and their source of water was either from the wells or taps, but stored in copper or brass vessels and so was the milk stored and boiled in them. It was observed that in this group of patients none were exclusively breastfed and all received animal milk at an earlier age as compared to other diseases.[9]

Subsequent comparisons between the feeding history of 10 children with ICC and 100 age, sex and caste matched controls from the same village, led to the hypothesis that ICC was a consequence of early introduction of animal milk feeds contaminated with copper from brass vessels.[10]

Usually, the brass vessels used for cooking are tinned from time-to-time, which can have a preventive role, but many households may not get the process done regularly due to the high expenses involved and continue to use them untinned. But gradually over a period of time, the use of these vessels has declined and very few rural households may still be found to use them.

Management

Management of ICC involves use of chelating agents like D pencilamine which unbinds copper from the cells. But it has been demonstrated that this may be beneficial only if it is given in the early stage of the disease when the child has not progressed to ascites or developed jaundice. Pencilamine is given in a dose of 20 mg/Kg/d, with or without prednisolone. The mortality rate was known to decline considerably after treatment to 53 percent as compared to 92 percent in a placebo group.[11]

With treatment, liver copper levels fall to near normal concentrations in contrast with persistently high liver copper concentrations in patients with Wilson's disease receiving pencilamine. This led to the hypotheses that although pencilamine was used to chelate copper from the bound form, its benefit was not necessarily a result of its removing excess copper or even detoxifying copper,[12] but could be due to an anti-inflammatory effect by inducing metallthionein, replacing glutathione or inhibiting collagen cross linking.[13]

Prevention

In view of the above mentioned evidence of copper deposition in the liver through copper/brass vessels, which are used for storing and boiling milk for infants, it seems but pertinent that prevention is the best cure for ICC, i.e. avoiding use of copper/brass vessels for heating or storing milk or water. This fact can be corroborated by a large intervention study in the Pune District of Maharashtra.[14] In this study, one group of population received an intensive program of health education, advising them against the use of brass utensils for preparation of infant feeds. It was observed that in this group of 4.1 million population, the use of brass vessels fell from 13 to 4 percent and the incidence of ICC declined to zero, where as in the control population of Ahmednagar of 2.7 million, the use of brass utensils and incidence of ICC also declined, probably due to the advice to the study group being percolated into this population too. But in Chandigarh where also this incidence had been reported, and the advice had not reached, the incidence did not change.[14]

Over a gradual period of time, due to change in lifestyle, brass vessels replaced stainless steel or hindalium vessels, which were increasingly getting popular. So, this change perhaps occurred spontaneously but gradually. Moreover, since brass vessels require more maintenance due to the tinning process (kallai), the availability of 'kallai vendors' also declined, who used to visit door to door to do the tinning of all brass vessels. Therefore, before brass vessels could completely be replaced by steel or other vessels, the availability of tinning became more expensive and less available. This led to an increase in the incidence of ICC before its decline, as it was phased out especially in the urban classes. Tinning is a process in which the uptake of copper is completely prevented from the by milk.[15]

A small percentage of the population however continue to use brass vessels even for boiling and storing milk, especially in the rural areas, which could be one reason why the incidence of ICC is still seen sporadically, especially in the referral hospitals.

REFERENCES

1. Robinson CH. Diet in disturbances of the liver, gallbladder and pancreas. In: Normal and Therapeutic Nutrition, 14th ed, Mac Millan Publishing Co. Inc. Oxford and IBH Publishing Co. 1972;483-93.
2. Silva IS, Perez RM, Oliveria PV, Cantagalo MI, Dantas E, et al. Iron overload and histopathological studies. J Gastroenterol Heptal 2005;20(2):243-8.
3. Sherlock S, Dolley J. Nutrition and metabolic liver disease. In: Diseases of the Liver and Biliary System 8th ed Oxford Medical Publication 1991;408-38.
4. Bianchi GP, Marchesini G, Fabbri A, et al. Vegetable vs. animal protein diet in cirrhotic patients with chronic encephalopathy. A randomized crossover comparison. J Intern Med 1993;233:385-92.
5. Charton CP, Buchanan E, Holder CE, et al. Intensive eneteral feeding in advanced cirrhosis: Reversal of malnutrition without precipitation of hepatic encephalopathy. Srch Dis Chil 1992;67:603-7.
6. Bavdekar A, Bhave S, Pandit A. Nutritional management in chronic liver disease. In J Ped Vol. 69, May 2002.

7. Portman B, Tanner MS, Mowet MP, Williams R. Orcein positive liver deposits in Indian Childhood Cirrhosis. Lancet 1978; 1: 1338-40.
8. Bhave S, Siddhaye D, Pradhan A, et al. Pediatric liver disease in India. Arch Dis Child 1982;57:922-8.
9. Tanner MS, Kantajian AH, Bhave SA, Pandit AN. Early introduction of copper contaminated animal milk feeds as a possible cause of Indian childhood cirrhosis. Lancet 1983;2:992-5.
10. Bhave SA, Pandit AN, Tanner MS. Comparison of feeding history of children with Indian childhood cirrhosis and paired controls. J Ped gastroenterol Nutr 1987;6:562-7.
11. Tanner MS, Bhave SA, Pradhan AM, Pandit AN. Clinical trials of pencilamine in Indian childhood cirrhosis. Arch Dis Child 1987;62:118-24.
12. Scheinberg IH, Sternleib I, Scholisky M, Stockert. Pencilamine may detoxify copper in Wilson's disease. Lancet 1987;2-95.
13. Mc Quaid A, Lamand M, Mason J. The interactions of pencilamine with copper in vivo and the effect on hepatic metallothionein levels and copper/zinc distribution: The implications for Wilson's disease and arthiritis therapy. J Lab Clin Med 1992;119:744-50.
14. Bhave SA, Pandit AN, Singh S, Walia BNS, Tanner MS. The prevention of Indian childhood cirrhosis. Ann Trop Pediatr 1992;12:23-30.
15. O'Neill NC, Tanner MS. Uptake of copper from brass utensils by bovine milk and its relevance to Indian childhood cirrhosis. J Pediatr Gastroenterol Nutr 1989; 9:167-72.

Chapter 16

Diet in Kidney Diseases

NEPHROTIC SYNDROME

Nephrotic syndrome (NS) is a disease primarily confined to the glomeruli. It is most commonly seen in children but can occur in adults too. In children, it is characterized by alterations of permselectivity at the glomerular capilliary wall, resulting in its ability to select the urinary loss of protein.

It is estimated that the annual incidence of nephritic syndrome ranges from 2-7 per 100,000 children and prevalence from 12-16 per 100,000.[1] There is epidemiological evidence of higher incidence of nephrotic syndrome in children from South Asia. In 95 percent of the cases, the condition is idiopathic. In less than 5 percent cases, the underlying causes could be systemic lupus erythematosus, amyloidosis and infection with HIV and hepatitis B and C virus.[2]

NS usually presenting in the first 3 months of life (congenital NS) could be secondary to intrauterine infections, e.g. congenital syphillus, toxoplasmosis and cytomegalovirus (CMV).

The classic definition of NS has been described as a clinical entity characterized by proteinuria, hypoalbuminemia and edema. The underlying physiological disturbance is an abnormal permeability of the glomerulus to macromolecules, resulting in increased filtered load of plasma proteins, part of which is reabsorbed and catabolized in the tubules, with the remainder appearing in the urine.[3]

Proteinuria in children is taken as 4 $mg/hr/m^2$ (166 mg/24 hrs/1.73 m^2).[4] In NS, it is generally associated with rates of protein >3.5 g/hr, but the International Study of Kidney Disease in Children (ISKDC), has defined proteinuria as excess of 40 mg $/hr/m^2$, equal to 1.66 g/24 hr/1.73 m^2, accompanied by hypoalbuminemia.[5] Protein losses in the urine are commonly 5-10 g/d and may exceed 30 g/d also.

Manifestation

Nephrotic syndrome is manifested by edema which may be generalized puffiness around the eyes, extremities, especially feet and ankles, swelling of the abdomen, facial swelling, foamy appearance of urine, weight gain due to fluid retention, anorexia and hypertension. In extreme cases, complications like hypertensive encephalopathy, congestive cardiac failure, electrolyte imbalance and acute renal failure may also occur.

DIETARY MODIFICATIONS IN NEPHROTIC SYNDROME

The objectives of dietary management are aimed at:

1. To maintain a state of good nutrition.
2. To control, or correct protein deficiency.
3. To prevent edema.
4. To provide palatable, easily digested meals as per individual needs.

A child with NS may require certain dietary modifications (including fluids) to be adhered to.

Fluids

Children with NS generally have problem regulating their water balance, which can cause edema. Therefore a restriction in fluids and sodium needs to be imposed. Fluids include any food which is liquid at room temperature. The fluid restriction includes insensible loss plus the previous day's output in conditions of oliguria, which is defined as urine output <1 ml/Kg/hr or 25 ml/Kg/d. Insensible loss of water is 400 $ml/m^2/d$.

It may be difficult for children to restrict fluid or water especially in hot temperate climates. Some useful tips with which the child can be helped to overcome thirst or the need to consume fluids are:

- Use of small glass/cups (standardized) to keep count of the intake
- Avoid salty foods as they increase thirst
- Iced tea and lemonade quench thirst better than fizzy drinks
- Frozen pieces of fruit (melon, grapes, and berries) can help quench thirst
- Chewing gum or hand candy can help quench thirst
- Rinsing of mouth
- Sucking a lemon wedge can stimulate saliva and moisten the mouth
- Staying away from sun can help avoid thirst in a child.

Proteins

Although there is excessive loss of protein in the urine, a high protein diet is contraindicated. The aim should be to replace the lost protein. Care should be taken to avoid high protein diets to prevent any tubular damage to the kidneys. A protein intake equivalent to the RDA for age is advisable which normally amounts to 1g/Kg body weight, to compensate for protein loss in the urine.

Sodium

The sodium content should be minimum to prevent fluid accumulation and edema. Foods generally high in sodium need to be restricted are:

- Salted wafers, popcorns, bakery products, snacks, chips, etc.
- Papads and pickles—all varieties
- Salted chutneys, sauces, commercial preparations e.g. soup cubes or powders
- Salted cashews, peanuts, savory and other dry fruits
- Commercial cheese, preservatives containing foods, noodle mixes and pasta
- Foods containing baking soda and ajino motto
- Salt to be avoided in cooking
- Generally 3-4 g/sodium per day is recommended, equivalent to about 2 g salt/d.

Since a day's normal diet contains about 1 g salt without adding during cooking, an added amount of 1 g for the whole day would make it 2 g of salt for the day's diet. To explain it simply, it would mean about 1/4th level tsp (5 g) to be distributed evenly for the whole day's diet which does not contain any salt while cooking.

Calories

Calories are recommended as for RDA, plus 10 percent extra for infections/illness.[5]

Potassium

Potassium is generally avoided during the phase of oliguria, which means restriction of fruits and fruit juices. All high protein feeds are also rich in potassium; therefore a balance has to be maintained, while selecting low potassium diets, at the same time adequate in proteins. Pulses are also rich in potassium, therefore need to be restricted. In case complications continue to persist, the sodium and potassium levels can be stabilized by peritoneal dialysis. A list of potassium rich foods to be avoided is listed in Table 16.1.[6]

ACUTE RENAL FAILURE (ARF)

Chronic glomerulonephritis, nephrosclerosis and pyelonephritis are some of the conditions which can lead to acute renal failure. Systemic lupus erythematosus (SLE) an autoimmune disorder involving the kidneys, acute tubular necrosis or dysplastic/contracted kidneys can also be precipitating factors in ARF. Other common causes in children could be dehydration, burns and snake bite.

Table 16.1: Potassium content of various indian foods

Low (< 100 mg)	*Moderate (100-200 mg)*	*High (>200 mg)*
Rice, suji, arrowroot flour peas, cucumber, radish pink, beetroot, broad beans, ridge gourd, snake gourd, tinda, fenugreek leaves tomato green, apple, banana ripe, guava, orange, papaya ripe, pine apple, pears, milk (buffalo).	Rice flakes, maize tender, wheat flour (refined), vermicelli, radish white, carrot, cauliflower, French beans, spinach, lichi, mango ripe, water melon, tomato ripe, pomegranate, cow's milk, liver (goat).	Wheat flour, maize dry, all pulses, colocasia, potato, sweet potato, tapioca, yam, brinjal, coconut, apricots, cherries, dates, lemon, sweet lime, mango, musk melon, plums, phalsa, chikoo, mutton (muscle), fish, prawn.

Ref. 6 (ICMR)

In this condition, the kidneys fail to maintain the normal composition of the blood. Some common terminologies referred to in this disease are:
Uremia: A condition arising from failure of kidney functions—literally meaning 'urine in the blood.'
Azotemia: Refers to accumulation of nitrogenous constituents in the blood.
Oliguria: Denotes scanty urine output (<0.5 ml/Kg/hr or <1 ml/Kg/hr in a neonate).
Anuria: Denotes urine production <100 ml/d.

In ARF, oliguria is usually present resulting in salt and water retention, catabolism and metabolic disturbances (low bicarbonate and calcium, high phosphate, potassium and urea).

The goal of dietary management in ARF should be:
- Prevent catabolism
- Maintain fluid and electrolyte balance
- Control metabolic abnormalities
- Aid recovery.

NUTRITIONAL MANAGEMENT

Children with ARF generally being in a state of catabolism are very anorexic and it is quite a challenge to get them to consume adequate diet. Moreover, there are quite a few restrictions imposed due to the limited amount of fluids to be given besides other protein and potassium rich foods.

Fluids

In short-term renal failure, the fluid load is restricted depending upon the urine output. In case oliguria continues to persist, peritoneal dialysis is initiated. By doing so, the diet restrictions, including fluids can be relaxed, considering the urine output plus the dialysate losses.

Proteins

Protein intake is restricted to 0.5 g/Kg/d, but with PD, it can be liberalized till 1.25 g/Kg/d. It would be advisable to provide high biological value proteins for optimum utilization.[7]

Calories

A high energy diet based on the RDA for age is recommended to make up for the catabolic state of the body.

Sodium

In condition of oliguria, no added salt is used in the diet, although it becomes a little difficult to make the child accept the diet. More varieties of sweet based foods can be offered spread over the day in smaller amounts.

The presence of hypertension in most of the children necessitates limiting sodium to <2 g/d. But in case, when PD has been started, sodium restriction may be relaxed to not more than 4 g/d. Though they are in a diuretic phase, caution still needs to be maintained and if required can be relaxed a little further, once the kidneys open up.

Potassium

During the oliguric phase, potassium is strictly restricted to control hyperphosphatemia, which implies restriction of all fruits and fruit juices. Once PD is on, this restriction may be relaxed. Table 16.2 highlights the plan for management of children with ARF.[7]

The choice of foods may be modified as per local availability, acceptance by the child and convenience of feeding, based on the exchange list of 3 gram portion size of various foods, as given in Table 16.3.

A policy plan for nutritional management or ARF has been highlighted in Fig. 16.1.[7]

Table 16.2: Dietary recommendations in acute renal failure

Volume	Depends on daily fluid removal (urine ± dialysate losses)
Energy	High to prevent catabolism
Protein	Low to prevent a high plasma urea, unless on prolonged peritoneal dialysis when a higher protein intake may be required
Salt	Low, except in the unusual circumstance of polyuric phase
Phosphate	Low to prevent hyperphosphatemia

Table 16.3: List of 3 g protein exchange of common foods

Foods	*Amount (g)*	*Serving size*
Rice	50	2 small
Chappati	25	1 small
Dal	12.5	½ small serving
Milk	100	3/4th tea cup
Bread	30	2 slices
Coconut, fresh	50	1 big cube
Potatoes	200	3-4 medium size
Beans	100	1 small serving
Peas, fresh	50	1 small serving

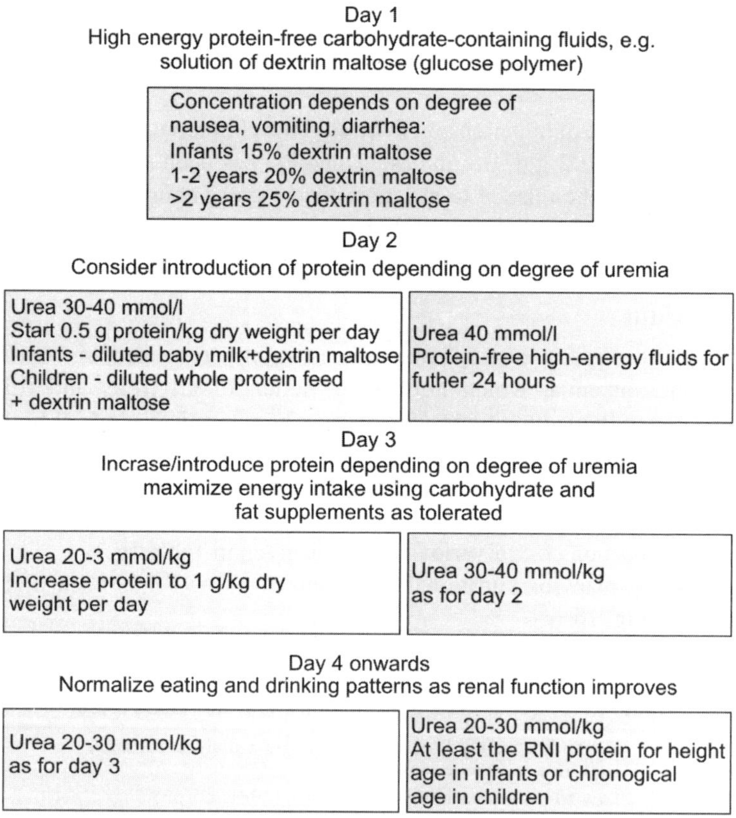

Fig. 16.1: Nutritional management of acute renal failure.
RNI = Reference nutrient intake.

CHRONIC RENAL FAILURE (CRF)

Chronic renal failure refers to a lon g standing progressive deterioration of renal functions. Symptoms develop slowly and include anorexia, nausea, vomiting, dysphagia, nocturia, lassitude, fatigue, decreased mental alertness, muscle twitching and cramps, water retention and undernutrition. Peripheral neuropathy and seizures may or may not be associated.

The National Kidney Foundation (NKF) has last updated the guidelines of the 2000 Kidney Disease Outcome Quality Initiative (KDOQI) in 2008, regarding the recommendations for dietary requirements of different nutrients.[8] They have graded the stages of chronic kidney disease (CKD) depending upon the rate of GFR (Table 16.4). The degree of GFR is standardized to the surface area (1.73 m^2) of a 70 Kg adult and is expressed as ml/min/1.73 m^2.

NUTRITIONAL MANAGEMENT

Management of children with chronic renal failure should aim at

- Reducing N intake
- Maintain N balance
- Cover essential amino acid requirement
- Provide adequate calories.

Energy

Oral intake of children with CRF is already compromised due to various associated factors like various factors like vomiting and anorexia, therefore spontaneous intake might be very inadequate. The recommended intake for in infants range from 100-120 Kcals/Kg/d, while for children, it would be 80-100 Kcals/Kg/d.

Table 16.4: NKF/KDOQI Classification for stages of CKD

Stage	*Description*	*GFR (ml/min/1.73m²)*	*Treatment*
One	Kidney damage with normal or increased GFR	≥90	1-5 T if kidney transplant recipient
Two	Kidney damage with mild or decreased GFR	60-90	
Three	Moderate with decreased GFR	30-59	
Four	Severe decreased GFR	15-29	
Five	Kidney failure	<15 (or dialysis)	5 D if dialysis (HD or PD)

Ref. 8: NKF/KDOQI Guidelines 2008

Protein

Protein requirement of a child in CRF is mainly based on the degree of glomerular filtration rate (GRF). A high protein intake poses a risk of aggravating acidosis, hyperkalemia and hyperphosphatemia, while on the other hand a restricted protein intake can help in reducing blood urea N (BUN), improve renal function and reduce symptoms of nausea, vomiting, muscle cramps and convulsions. Certain authors have based the protein requirements of children with CRF by broadly classifying them into mild, moderate and severe CRF as shown in Table 16.5.[5]

In case of young children, as they begin to take more proteins from solids, milk products may need to be restricted. About 70 percent of proteins should be from high biological value sources, e.g. milk and milk products, fish or cheese. But, due to the high phosphate content of these, even such products may need to be given with caution. The balance of proteins can be given in the form of lower biological value protein sources, e.g. rice, pasta, bread and potatoes, which can be used liberally.

Fluids

The amount of fluids allowed will depend upon the extent of water retention. Mostly, that is taken care of by giving diuretics and restricting sodium. In case of failure to still achieve this, dialysis may be considered.

Sodium

The amount of sodium is equally restricted to take care of hypertension (if existing), and fluid retention. Salt intake can be maintained at 30-600 mg/d in infants and 1-2 g/d in older children.[5]

Potassium

Potassium levels are generally restricted in case of hyperkalemia (>6.5 mmol/l), which may involve restricting of fruits and green vegetables like potatoes, though low in proteins, are a fairly good source of potassium, therefore, these may be incorporated in the diet by soaking and discarding the water. This process allows a considerable amount of potassium

Table 16.5: Protein requirements of children with CRF dased on GFR

Type of GFR	*Proteins g/Kg*		
	0-1 year	*1-5 years*	*5-10 years*
Mild (GFR 20-40)	1.8	1.4	1
Moderate (GFR 5-20)	1.4	1.0	0.8
Severe (GFR <5)	1	0.8	0

Ref. 5 (International study of kidney disease in children, 1998)

Table 16.6: Diet for a child with renal failure sample MENU (Base diet)

Breakfast	
Sweet sago porridge (sago—25-30 g + sugar—10-15 g)	1 serve
Mid Morning	
Baked potatoes (with butter optional)	50-75 g
Lunch	
Rice	1 serve (25-30 g)
Chappati/Parantha	1 medium (25 g)
Curd	100 g
Evening	
Sago vada, sweet (sago—50 g, sugar—10-15 g)**	1-2 pcs.
Dinner	
Rice, plain/fried	1 serving (25 g)
Vegetables+potato mix	1-2 serving (100-200 g)
Sago, sweet	1 serving (25 g)

Note: *Milk may be used instead of curd.
**Potatoes may be used with sago to make the vada.
Fruit may be added in the menu if potassium not restricted.

to be leeched out. In fact even other green vegetables should be prepared by leeching out the water after soaking them in water for a few hours. In case if potassium levels drop, as hypokalemia may also occur in between, liberal amounts of fruit juice may be offered besides giving potassium supplement (Pot Chlor) if required. A sample diet for a child with renal failure may be based on the pattern as shown in Table 16.6.

If proteins are to be increased, equivalent exchange of protein (3 g) may be suitably added (Table 16.3).

To increase calories, 1-2 exchanges of oil/sugar may be added as required.

Calories: 1000-1100 Proteins: 8-10 g
Sodium: <100 mg Potassium: <20 mEq

DIALYSIS

Patients with chronic renal disease who fail to respond to conventional management may require dialysis to maintain renal functions to near normal levels.

Energy Requirements

Children with chronic kidney disease (CKD) generally have poor intake, especially those in stages 2-5 D due to reduced appetite and vomiting. Supplemental nutritional support is recommended where the usual intake of a child with CKD stages 2-5 D (Table 16.5) fails to meet the recommended dietary intake.

Early intervention is essential with introduction of tube feeds, if energy requirement cannot be met orally. A small percentage of children may have excessive energy intake, therefore dietary intervention and lifestyle changes are needed to tackle the long-term complications of obesity. The recommended energy intake as per the NKF/KDOQI Pediatric Guidelines (last updated in 2008), for stages 2-5 and 5 D have recommended 100 percent of the estimated requirement for dialytic protein and amino acid losses. Based on the response in rate of weight gain or loss, suitable adjustments can be made. However, it has been recommended that tube fed children and infants be encouraged to continue some oral intake or have continued oral stimulation, e.g. sucking or a pacifier and/or positive non-threatening contact with food.[8] Advanced CKD stages are often associated with anorexia and gastrointestinal disorders, which may inhibit the ability to maintain adequate nutritional status through oral and/or enteral nutrition.

Fats, carbohydrates and proteins may be substituted for one another to meet the energy needs. Uneven distribution of calories from each of the macronutrients may be associated with an increased risk of some chronic diseases like coronary heart disease, obesity and diabetes mellitus, which are commonly seen in children with CKD over a certain length of time. Therefore, the acceptable macronutrient distribution (AMDR) in children with CKD should be as given as in Table 16.7.[9]

The use of protein supplements are recommended to augment the inadequate oral and/or enteral protein intake in children in stages 2-5 and 5 D of CKD, as these children are unable to meet their requirements orally.

Poor appetite and vomiting are the frequent problems seen in children with CKD and this is the main reason for their poor intake. Vomiting and irritability are along with discomfort are suggestive of gastroesophageal reflux (GER) initially can be managed by concentrated feeds to reduce the volume and increase the density, and maintaining elevated position after feeds.[10] Tube feeding is a suitable alternative under such conditions, which may be initiated by small frequent feeding. This can help achieve significant weight gain and catch up growth.[11]

Table 16.7: Acceptable macronutrient distribution range (AMDR) in children with CKD

Macronutrients	*1-3 years*	*4-10 years*
Carbohydrates	45-65%	45-65%
Fats	30-40%	25-30%
Proteins	5-20%	10-30%

(Ref. 6)

The AMDR ranges for a healthy distribution of calories from carbohydrates, fats and proteins are based upon the evidence that consumption of greater or lesser than these ranges may be associated with nutrient inadequacy and increased risk of developing such chronic diseases as coronary heart disease, obesity, diabetes and/or cancer.

Generally calorie dense formulae are prescribed for infants, but since there are no AMDR guidelines for children under 1 year, care should be taken that when increasing the caloric density of the formula, the distribution of proteins, fats and carbohydrates should be kept consistent with the base formula,[12] which must adhere to strict standards (7 to 12 percent proteins, 40 to 54 percent fats and 36 to 56 percent carbohydrates).

Protein Requirements

Although there is no evidence for dietary protein restriction to maintain a nephroprotective effect, it can be restricted safely to 0.8-1.1 g/kg/d in children with CKD. This will help reduce the accumulation of nitrogenous waste products and facilitate lowering of dietary phosphorous levels. It will also help delay the onset of signs and symptoms of uremia. The Committee of the KDOQI, 2008 felt that implementation and maintenance of a strict low protein diet requires a major life style change and hence not very practical and acceptable by many families. Therefore, moderate protein restriction aiming at 100 to 140 percent of the RDA in CKD stage 3 and 100 to 120 percent of the RDA in CKD stages 4-5 as given in Table 16.8 may be a reasonable compromise in most cases.[8]

These protein recommendations refer to a stable child, assuming that energy intake will result in inefficient utilization of proteins, with increased production of urea.

In children with CKD stage 5 D, it is recommended to maintain the dietary intake at 100 percent of the RDA, for ideal body weight, plus an allowance for dialytic protein and amino acids.

Vitamins and Trace Element Requirements

Patients with CKD and those on dialysis therapy are at an increased risk of vitamin and mineral deficiency due to abnormal renal metabolism, inadequate intake and poor gastrointestinal absorption and dialysis relayed to losses.

The recommendations for various B complex vitamins (B_1), riboflavin (B_2), niacin (B_3), pantothenic acid (B_5), pyridoxine (B_6), biotin, cobalamin, ascorbic acid, retinol and tocopherol, vitamin K, folic acid, copper and zinc for children with CKD stages 2 to 5 and 5D.

Table 16.8: Recommended dietary protein intake in children with CKD stages 3-5 and 5 D

Age	*Dietary reference intake (DRI)*				
	DRI g/Kg/d	*Recommended for CKD Stage 3 g/Kg/d 100-140 % RDA*	*Recommended for CKD stage 4-5 g/Kg/d 100-120 % RDA*	*Recommended for HD g/kg/d*	*Recommended for PD g/Kg/d*
0-6 months	1.5	1.5-2.1	1.5-1.8	1.6	1.8
7-12 months	1.2	1.2-1.7	1.2-1.5	1.3	1.5
1-3 years	1.05	1.05-1.5	1.05-1.25	1.15	1.3
4-13 years	0.95	0.9-1.35	0.95-1.15	1.05	1.1
14-18 years	0.85	0.85-1.2	0.85-1.05	0.95	1.0

Ref. 8 (NKF/KDOQI guidelines 2008)

In case dietary protein is not achieved at 100 percent of the RDA, it is suggested that supplementation of vitamins and trace elements be provided or if there is clinical evidence of a deficiency of any of these vitamins. For children with CKD 5 D on dialysis, a water soluble vitamin supplement is recommended.

Calcium needs to be supplemented for children with CKD stages 2-5 and 5 D from nutritional sources and phosphate binders in the range of 100-200 of the DRI.

Fluid and Electrolyte Requirements

In children with CKD, the requirement of fluids and electrolytes varies according to the status of the kidney disease, degree of residual kidney function and type of renal replacement therapy. The sodium and potassium restriction or supplementation depends upon the volume of urine output, ability to concentrate urine hydration status and the presence or absence of hypertension or hyperkalemia. The KDOQI recommendations for children with CKD are:

1. Supplemental free water and sodium supplements should be considered for children with CKD stages 2-5 and 5 D and polyurea to avoid chronic intravascular depletion and to promote optimal growth.
2. For all infants with CKD stage 5 D, on peritoneal dialysis, sodium supplements should be considered.
3. Children and infants with CKD stages 2-5 and 5 D, who are hypertensive, restriction of sodium should be advised.
4. For infants with CKD stage 5 D on peritoneal dialysis (PD) therapy sodium supplements need to be prescribed.
5. For children with oliguria, fluid intake is advised to prevent complications of fluid overload.
6. Children with hyperkalemia, need to be advised potassium restriction, especially those with CKD stages 2-5 and 5 D.

NUTRITIONAL MANAGEMENT IN TRANSPLANT PATIENTS

Children, who have undergone renal transplantation, need to be monitored and assessed for their growth and development to meet their nutritional requirements while minimizing the side effects of immune suppressive drugs.

Management of the child with kidney transplant includes care of the graft besides care of complications of CKD stages 1-5 T. They continue to require dietary modifications posttransplant. The modifications include in terms of hypertension, hyperkalemia, hypophosphatemia, hypomagnesmia and hyperglycemia, which could be complication of immunosuppressive drugs. For children with CKD stages 2-5 T, management of protein and phosphorous is done as for children with similar GFRs before transplantation.

The energy requirement of children with CKD stages 1-5 T should be equal to 100 percent of the estimated energy requirements (EER) adjusted for BMI. Adjustments in view of loss or gain in weight can be done as per requirement.

A balance of calories from carbohydrates, proteins and unsaturated fats within the physiological ranges recommended by AMDR of the DRI is suggested for children with CKD stages 1-5 T to prevent or manage obesity, dyslipidemia and corticosteroid induced diabetes.

Children with CKD stages 1-5 T and hypertension or abnormal serum electrolytes concentrations which are common with immunosuppressive drugs need to be managed by suitable dietary modifications.

Calcium and vitamin D intakes need to be provided at least 100 percent of the DRI for children with CKD 1-5 T, however, not exceeding 200 percent of the DRI.[6]

Fluids including water and other beverages should not be sweetened with simple sugars, to avoid excess weight gain, hyperglycemia and dental decay.

Food hygiene and safety and avoidance of foods from doubtful sources need to be ensured strictly for immunosuppressed children with CKD stages 1-5 T.

REFERENCES

1. Eddy AA, Symons JM. Nephrotic syndrome in childhood. Lancet 2003; 362:629-39.
2. Mc Kinney PA, Feltbower RG, Brocklebank JT, Fitzpatric MM. Time, trends and ethnic patterns of childhood nephritic syndrome in Yorkshire, UK. Pediatr Nephrol 2001;16:1040-4.
3. Trompeter RS and barret TM. Treatment and management of nephritic syndrome in children. In: The nephritic syndrome Eds. Cameron JS and Glassock RJ (1988).
4. Barret TH. Renal Disorders. In: Clayton BE, Round JM Eds. Chemical Pathology and the Sick Child, Oxford: Blackwell Scientific Publications 1984;120-43.
5. International Study of kidney Disease in Children. Nephrotic syndrome in children: Prediction of histopathology from clinical and laboratory characterstics at time of diagnosis. Kidney Int. 1998; 13:159-65.
6. Gopalan C, Rama Sastri BV, Balasbramanian SC. Nutritive Value of Indian Foods, National Institute of Nutrition, ICMR, Hyderabad, 2002.

7. Rees L, Webb N, Brogan p (Eds): Acute Renal Failure In: Pediatric Nephrology, Oxford University Press, 2007;360-84.
8. NKF/KDOQI Clinical Practice Guideline for Nutrition in Children with Chronic Kidney Disease: 2008 Update. Am J Kidney Dis. 53:S1-S124 (Suppl 2), 2009.
9. NKF/KDOQI Clinical Practice Guideline for Nutrition in Children with Chronic Kidney Disease: 2008 Update. Am J Kidney Dis. 53:S1-S124 (Suppl 2), 2009.
10. Dello Strologo L, Principato F, Sinibaldi D, et al. Feeding dysfunction in infants with severe chronic renal failure after long-term nasogastric feeding. Pediatr Nephrol 1997;11:84-6.
11. Rudolph CD, Mazur LJ, Liptak GS, et al. Guidelines for evaluation and treatment of gastroesophageal reflux in infants and children. Recommendations of the North American Society for Pediatric Gastroenterology and Nutrition. J Ped Gastroenterol Nutr 2001 (Suppl 2) 32:S1-31.
12. Spinozzi NS, Nelson PA. Nutrition support in the new born intensive care unit. J Ren Nutr 1996;188-97.

Chapter 17 Enteral Nutrition in Hospitalized Patient

Enteral nutrition (EN) is an alternative method of providing nutrition support to a patient who is otherwise unable or not in a condition to receive oral nutrition. In a child it becomes all the more essential that nutritional support is provided where there is inadequate oral intake or the child is very malnourished and unable to ingest the required amount of feeds orally. This nutrition support can be provided through the enteral route where the gut is intact. EN goes a long way in restoring the nutritional status of the child and plays an adjunctive role in the disease and immune process. It improves physical and mental functions, decreases the effect of catabolism and prevents further weight loss.

Feeding by the enteral route may reduce sepsis, blunt the hypermetabolic response to trauma and maintain gut integrity.[1] It is recommended that a child with malnutrition or likely to receive inadequate nutrient intake for a minimum of 7 days or more, should be offered EN.

EN has been successfully used within 24-48 hours after surgery or trauma to provide fluids, electrolytes and nutritional support. In case there is gastric ileus, nasogastric feeding can be replaced by nasojejeunal or nasointestinal feeding. This allows successful post pyloric passage of the feeds (Kudsk, 1994)

EN formulae can vary in composition and nutrient density. By and large these include standard whole protein formulae, elemental or peptide based or any disease specific formulations. These may also include certain specific nutrients like glutamine, arginine and omega-3fatty acids. Apart from these indigenously formulates feeds vcan also be administered by modifying the locally available commercial protein or MCT based formulae to the indigenous formulation (Kitchen based) have also been successful in the developing countries. This can help in reducing the cost in an otherwise resource limited setting.

According to the British Medical Association (BMA), it is important to identify the need for enteral feeding, before deciding whether a child should be artificially fed.[2]

INDICATIONS FOR EN SUPPORT IN CHILDREN

EN support may be used for children in any of the following conditions:

Unable to suck/swallow, e.g. in ventilated patients.

Swallowing may be unsafe, e.g. in cerebral palsy, seizures.

Poor sucking, e.g. in premature infants.

Increased requirements, e.g. in conditions of cystic fibrosis, burns, trauma or any congenital heart disease.

Poor appetite secondary to illness like in disorders of the liver, kidney or cancer.

Congenital abnormalities, e.g. in tracheoesophageal fistula, orofacial malformation.

Unpalatability of specialized feeds, e.g. Crohn's disease.

Continuous supply of nutrients required to prevent hypoglycemia or in glycogen storage disease type 1.

Once the decision to provide nutrition entrerally is made, the patient needs to be explained regarding the objective of doing so. This can be done by explaining the proposed benefits of the treatment, i.e. weight gain, speedy recovery and prevention of starvation explaining the possible risks and complications involved, e.g. infection, granulation, gastroesophageal reflux, tube displacement, leakage, vomiting, retching, diarrhea or constipation or blocked tube, explaining the impact of the treatment on the family, e.g. restricted freedom of mobility, monitoring of feeds and checking for aspirates.

Nutritional Requirements in EN

Calories

The nutritional requirements can be calculated based on the RDA for age, as is done when planning an oral feeding. However, for bedside calculation, a minimum requirement may be determined which may be adequate for an average child. The formula used is 100 calories/kg up to 1 year, 1000 calories at 1 year and thereafter, 1000 +10 calories/each year up to puberty. At puberty, the requirement is equated to 1 unit of energy (2,400 calories).[3]

Proteins

The protein requirement can be calculated as 10-15 percent of the calories, which amounts to 1.5-2 g/kg/d. In case the child is very malnourished, protein may be increased gradually to 3-4 g/kg/d. In conditions of renal failure, the protein may be decreased to around 0.5 g/kg/d. The protein requirement may be met by utilizing either whole proteins, protein hydrolysates or as individual amino acids or a combination of these based on their absorptive capacity, requirement and tolerance. Whole proteins being less expensive can be given in patients with no suspected major absorptive defect or protein allergy. These also allow greater nutrient density. In patients who are able to tackle whole proteins or have any specific absorptive defect or deficiency, can be offered protein hydrolysate. However, hydrolyzed proteins have high osmolar load as compared to the whole proteins

Fats

The high caloric density of fats (especially triglycerides) makes it a highly desirable nutrient in the nutritional support of the hospitalized child. Three major considerations are involved in the use of dietary fats- the use and absorption of LCT, MCT and the requirement for EFA.

It has been recommended that if there are no defects in the absorption of fats, the choice should be LCT. Excessive use of MCT in patients with intact mechanisms can lead to osmotic diarrhea due to the rapid hydrolysis of MCT to free fatty acids and glycerol. A combination of LCT and MCT fats may be justified in order to gain maximal absorption in patients in whom increased calories are vital.[4] A total of 25-30 percent of calories can be provided by fats out of which up to 10-15 percent of the fats can be provided as visible fat. In case where there is suspected fat malabsorption, MCT can be provided as a safe source of fat, e.g. in conditions of hepatobiliary diseases.

Carbohydrates

Ideally 50-60 percent of the energy can be provided by carbohydrates. In diseases involving the mucosa of the small intestine, all of the disaccharides may be depressed. Lactase is one of the most sensitive to injury and the last to recover too. This may result in transient lactase deficiency. Starvation by itself is known to depress the disaccharide activity, therefore it is important to avoid or minimize dietary sources of lactose in treating the malnourished child.

Micronutrients

Since children who are malnourished with their intake compromised, there is an increased demand for all micronutrients, especially during the acute phase of illness. Supplementing these with the enteral feeds should be done as per the recommended doses.

Properties of an Enteral Feed

Enteral feeds although are formulated to provide more or less complete nutritional requirements, certain factors need to be kept in mind regarding their effects on the patient (Table 17.1).[4]

Physiologic Effects

The effects of various types of food or acid secretion are proportionate primarily to the protein content. There is evidence to suggest that the carbohydrate fraction of the meal stimulates gastrin secretion. When amino acids are administered as mixtures, as in the defined formula diets, pancreatic stimulation occurs. This can be averted, if the feeds are given intrajejunally and at a neutral pH. This kind of therapy is particularly suitable in case of patients with fistulae or pancreatitis.

Table 17.1: Special considerations in administering feeds through enteral route

Risk of aspiration
Comatose patient
Restrained patient
Small Infant
Depressed gag reflex
Palatability
Distorted N: calorie ratio
Inappropriate formulations
Osmolality-formulae with increased nutrient intensity.

Refer. 4.

Nitrogen: Calorie Ratio

Generally the protein content of enteral feeds is 15-17 percent of the energy content. In such a case the N: Calorie ratio is approximately 1:150, which is considered adequate for recovery and growth in infants suffering from varying degrees of malnutrition. However, in cases requiring unusually high protein content due to excessive losses, higher protein ratio also can be provided for maintenance.

Uniformity

Defined enteral diets are designed to be uniform in composition and this is the reason it can be used as a supplement to total parenteral nutrition. These formulae are devoid of fiber as a result of which there is a decrease in stool frequency, weight and bulk and the stools are usually dark green in color, watery and nonformed.

Osmolality

An important factor to be considered when choosing or formulating an enteral formula is the osmolality of the feed. An osmolality above

600 mOsm/l can lead to an increased incidence of gastrointestinal symptoms and intolerance to feeds. It has been shown that an osmolality of 560 mosm/l can cause a significant delay in gastric emptying.[4]

Carbohydrates electrolytes and amino acids are the major factors determining the gastrointestinal osmotic load of a formula. Smaller particles like glucose and free amino acids contribute to a higher osmolality than do larger particles such as polysaccharides or intact protein molecules. That is why hydrolyzed proteins and monosaccharides will tend to have a higher osmolality than will formula with intact protein and glucose polymers.[5]

An osmolality of less than 460 mOsm/kg has been recommended for infant formula, therefore for children younger than 4 years, the enteral formula should be <400 mOsm/Kg and for older ones, <600 mOsm/Kg.[6,7]

Contraindications of Enetral Nutrition

Contraindications to enteral feeding in most cases are relative and rather than absolute. It is also dependent upon the appropriate feeding site, administration technique, formula and equipment.

Terminal illness: Potential problems include aspiration, diarrhea, overhydration, discomfort and cost.

Short bowel: Patients with a short bowel often require TPN for 1-3 months postsurgery, while the remaining bowel adapts to allow adequate nutrient absorption. Adaptation of the gut is accelerated by early institution of some enteral feeding.

Obstruction: Complete mechanical obstruction of the GI below the duodenum or pseudo-obstruction like in GI motility disorders can be contraindication for EN.

GI bleeding: Chronic, slow upper GI bleed may not be an absolute contraindication for EN but frequent vomiting or nausea may require withholding of EN temporarily. In such cases, small bowel feedings rather than gastric feeding are a better option.

Vomiting and diarrhea: Vomiting may make it difficult to maintain the nasogastric feeding tube in place, in which case small bowel feeding can be done. Diarrhea may not be due to EN but could be associated with the type of feeding formula, e.g. lactose based or medications received as in case of antibiotics.

GI ischemia: GI ischemia may result due to the disease state itself or medical treatment which may reduce the blood flow to the gut, e.g.

critically ill patients with a low cardiac output, patients with sepsis and those with multiorgan failure.

Ileus: In surgical conditions like perforation, anastomatic leaks, intra-peritoneal hemorrhage, peritonitis and other intra-abdominal infections, ileus can occur. This is more frequently known to affect the stomach and large bowel. Therefore to overcome this hurdle postpyloric feeding tube placement can be done.

GI inflammation: In conditions like IBD (Inflammatory Bowel Disease), radiation or chemotherapy, inflammation or enteritis is commonly seen. In such cases, bowel rest is advised and parenteral nutrition may be resorted to. Bowel rest is advised in pancreatitis, although successful enteral nutrition support has been demonstrated to yield good results.

Routes of EN

After deciding upon the type of enteral nutrition to be administered, the next step is to evaluate the way to do it. Ideally 'where the gut works, it should be used.' Oral feeding whenever, possible even though in small proportions must be preferred to maintain the gut integrity. Breastfeeding if possible should be continued. But in cases where oral intake is not possible due to various reasons like swallowing difficulty, esophageal atresia, gastrectomy, seizures or other neurological conditions, alternative route of feeding have to be made use of. This will depend upon the best available route and feasibility of administration at the available site. Some common routes used are:

- Nasogastric
- Nasojejunal
- Gastrostomy/Jejunostomy

Nasogastric Feeding (NG Feeding)

This is the most preferred route used in most children with intact GIT or who are unable to swallow orally. The nasogastric feedings are used mainly for short-term use (6-8 weeks). Formula or kitchen based feeds are generally given through this route either as bolus feeds at periodic intervals or as continuous drip method. The latter is a better option and acceptable since there is better tolerance as compared to bolus feeding. The rule is to begin with small feeds at periodic intervals and gradually increase the volume and density of the feeds as the tolerance improves. A common observation is that in case of malnourished children, who are unable to eat orally as per the required dose, if NG feeding is initiated and continued for a few days, the appetite of the child begins to improve and gradually they can be weaned off the NG feed completely. However, NG feeding is contraindicated in patients with seven esophagitis or who have no obstruction between the nose and stomach.

Nasojejunal Feeding (NJ Feeding)

This method of feeding involved placement of the tube well beyond the stomach, into the jejunum, so that, the feed is deposited beyond the pylorus, thus preventing regurgitation. This route is used typically for children who are at risk of aspiration which include diminished gag reflex, delayed gastric emptying, frequent vomiting or severe gastro-esophageal reflux (GER). The intestinal wall having a larger surface area allows for rapid absorption of iso and hyposmolar solutions. Some problems of pain, nausea, distension or hypomotility and diarrhea may result if the formula is hyperosmolar, has whole protein sources, complex carbohydrates and LCTs. Necrotising enterocolitis is one complication which could be related to use of hyperosmolar solutions in premature infants.[4]

Gastrostomy Feedings

Gastrostomy feeding is used in children expected to be on long-term NG feeding, e.g. in severe neurological impairment, esophageal pathology or severe cardiorespiratory disease, who have an intact GIT. The rate and volume of feeding is done as is done in NG feeding. In conditions where the stomach or duodenum integrity is affected, jejunostomy feeding tube is used. The considerations for using this route are same as for NJ feeding.

Methods of Administration of EN

The mode of feed delivery is based on the condition of the patient and the anatomic location of the tube (gastric or transpyloric). The feeds may be delivered either through intermittent bolus or continuous drip method. Intermittent bolus feeds are given 2-4 hourly over a period of 15-20 minutes by gravity, while continuous drip method involves infusion of nutrients at a constant rate over several hours. The choice of the type of delivery mode depends on a number of factors like:

- Enteral access route
- Volume of feed required
- Stability of the patient
- Gastrointestinal tolerance of the feed
- Age of the patient
- Type of formula

Nutrient requirements
Patient cooperation and mobility

Initiation of Advancement of Feeding

The rate of advancement of enteral feeding is contingent on the structure and function of the patients GIT. Children being weaned from PN to enteral nutrition or who are malnourished may require a more conservative feeding progression than what is typically administered to children with normal GI.

General Considerations

There are a certain general guidelines to be considered when advancing enteral nutrition in children, which have been laid down based on institutional practices and modifications of adult regimens as under:

Plan for a 2-5 day period to meet the nutritional goals

Use isotonic feedings initially.

Avoid making a simultaneous change in volume and concentration.

Use of dilute feedings in patients with altered GI functions or when weaning from PN to EN.

Advance continuously and gradually in very critical or malnourished children.

Increase volume before increasing concentration when administering transplyloric feeds.

Advance concentration before volume when administering gastric feeds.

If not tolerated, revert back to the last tolerated concentration and volume and progress slowly again.

Continuous Drip Feeding

Begin at a rate of 1-2 ml/Kg/h.

Advance in increment of 0.5-1 ml/Kg/h every 8-24 hours.

Rate of feeding for various age groups as recommended (Table 17.2).

Intermittent Feeding

Determine the total volume of formula needed to provide nutritional goal.

Begin delivery at 25 percent of the volume goal on the first day.

Space the formula volume equally between 6-8 feedings.

Increase formula volume by 25 percent as tolerated, with total volume equally divided between numbers of feedings.

Administer by gravity over 15-30 minutes.

Table 17.2: Recommended rate of continuous drip feeding for children

Age	*Weight (kg)*	*Initial rate (ml/h)*	*Max. Rate (ml/h)*
Infants	3-10	3-10	25-50
Toddler/Pre-school	10-20	10-20	60-70
School age	20-40	20-40	80-100
Adolescent	> 40	40-50	100-150

The general considerations for advancing the enteral nutrition in children have been laid down,[8] which are based on institutional practices and modification of adult regimen as follows:

Complications of EN

Although administration of EN through tube feeding takes care of all the nutrient requirements of the patient and feeding can be ensured even when the child is sick or unable to take orally, there are certain factors to be borne in mind while administering EN, which if not considered may lead to complications. Some of the common complications known to occur while giving feeds are:

Mechanical Complications

Tube displacement: These may involve placement of the feeding tube which could be displaced or faulty placement resulting in lacerations along the esophagus, upper airway injury, GI injuries, bleeding ulcers, extrusion or migration of feeding tubes. Many of these problems occur with larger or stiffer tubes and can be minimized by using small bore feeding tubes and meticulous nursing care.

Tube clogging: This can occur with feeds which are protein based and viscous in nature. Mostly kitchen based feeds may tend to have some residue settling down is likely to clog which passing through the tube. Flushing of the tube with water after every feed or checking of aspirate can minimise the problem.

Aspiration: This is a serious complication of any enteral feeding. Aspiration pneumonia can occur in 5 percent of gastric fed patients, resulting in cough, bronchospasm, pulmonary edema, pneumonia, empyema and respiratory failure.[9,10]

GI Complications

GER: Reflux of contents from the stomach can occur in some patients when the gastric pressure exceeds that of the pressure of the lower esophageal stricture (LES) which prevents the gastric contents from volume or ascites (due to the increased abdominal pressure), reflux can be encountered.

Diarrhea: Diarrhea can be frequently seen in patients receiving enteral feeds. This could be either if feed is lactose based (e.g. in high volume milk based feeds) or could also be due to bacterial growth or presence of toxins, or medications, e.g. certain antibiotics, SBS, high fat based feeds or due to the nature of the disease itself. Withdrawal of feeding is not recommended in such cases, but a change of formula or tackling the infective source could help minimize the complication. In extreme cases, if no specific cause can be elicited for the problem, enteral feeds may be considered to be replaced by parenteral nutrition.

Constipation: This can result from inactivity, decreased small bowel motility, decreased fluid intake, impaction or lack of dietary fiber. Adequate hydration and use of fiber based formulae can help minimize the problem. Laxatives and enemas may also help relieve the problem.

Metabolic Complications

Hyperglycemia: This is not a very common problem because of enteral feeding, but could be encountered in patients who may be diabetic. At times high carbohydrate feeds may also cause increased blood sugar levels. Patient on IV fluids over a considerable period when fed enterally also may develop hyperglycemia. Increased blood glucose levels should be tackled immediately by use of insulin. The aim should be to maintain the blood glucose concentrations below 150-180 mg/d.

Electrolyte and mineral deficiencies: Losses of electrolytes (sodium, potassium) through stools, ostomies, fistulae, urine and skin can result in considerable electrolyte and animal losses too. Mineral deficiencies like magnesium, calcium, phosphorous might also be encountered along with the above problems, coupled with lack of these minerals in the eneteral feeds. Adequate supplementation of these needs to be considered in such cases.

Refeeding syndrome: This is a condition known to occur in malnourished children, where there are acute intracellular shifts of electrolytes or cell anabolism is stimulated.[11]

Vitamin deficiencies: Both water soluble and fat soluble vitamin deficiencies can be encountered in patients on EN. Children with pancreatic enzyme deficiency, e.g. in cystic fibrosis are prone to be deficient in vitamin A, D and E as these require bile and pancreatic enzymes for absorption. Other conditions where such deficiencies can occur are in malabsorption. These vitamins need to be monitored and replaced along with the EN. Similarly among the water soluble vitamins are folate and ascorbic acid and thiamine, which could be deficient in the enteral feeds and may need adequate replacement.

Dehydration: Dehydration is commonly encountered among patients on enteral feeds. An average requirement of water is 1 ml/calorie consumed. The use of concentrated formulae or high protein feeds may result in decrease in fluids, e.g. loss of body fluids when there is urea dieresis with high protein feeds. Restoration of intravascular volume and water balance can reverse this condition.

REFERENCES

1. Directors ASfPaENASPENBo. Guidelines for use of Parenteral and Enteral Nutrition in adult and pediatric patients. JPEN 1993;17(4);1-52.
2. Dartford and Gravesham NHS Trust and Dartford Gravesham and Swanley Primary Care Trust. Jan 2007, Pediatric Enteral Feeding Guidelines Operational Policy (Infants and Children).
3. K.E. Elizabeth. Enteral Nutrition and Parenteral Nutrition. In: Nutrition and Child Development. Paras Medical Publishers 3rd eds. 2004;3:188-217.
4. Robert M Suskind, Leiko NS, Murray C and Munro HN. Enteral Suport of the hospitalized child. In: Textbook of Pediatric Nutrition. Ed. Raven Press, New York, 1981; 352-74.
5. Nancy Nevin Folino and Murna Miller. Enteral Nutrition. In: Handbook of Pediatric Nutrition. Patricia Queen Samour, Kathy King Helm and Carol E. Lang. Jones and Bartlett Publishers, Massachusetts, 2nd eds. 2004;2:513-49.
6. Kalawitter BM. Pediatric Nutrition Support. In: Williams CP, ed. Pediatric Manual of Clinical Dietetics. Chicago IL: The Am Dietet Assoc 1998.
7. Cox JH, Nutrition Manual for At-Risk Infants and toddlers. Chicago IL: Precept Press ed. 1997.
8. Lingard CD. Enteral Nutrition. In: Handbook of Pediatric Nutrition, Queen PM and Lang CE. Ed. 1993, Aspen Publishers. Inc.
9. Hamaai E. Gastroesophageal reflex during gastostomy feeding. JPEN 1995;19:172-73.
10 Gustke RF, Varma RR, Soegel KH. Gastric reflux during perfusion of the proximal small bowel. Gastroenterology 1970;59:890-95.
11. Solomon SM, Kirby DF. The Refeeding syndrome: A review. JPEN,14: 90-7.

Chapter 18 Nutritional Support of the Critically Ill Child

Adequate nutrition is an important aspect of management of a critically ill child. The outcome of a child in the critical phase is largely dependent upon the appropriate nutritional support (nor too less nor excess) and has the potential to reverse or reduce adverse long-term consequences. Patients most likely to benefit from nutritional support are those with baseline malnutrition in whom a protracted period of starvation would otherwise occur. In well-nourished children with short (<1 week) anticipated duration of nil by mouth feeding, improvement in nutritional status may be difficult to demonstrate.

Indications for nutritional support in the critically ill child include pre-existing malnutrition, excessive metabolic demands and the inability to ingest nutrients for prolonged periods.

Nutritional management of the critical ill child involves:

- Assessment
- Administration
- Monitoring.

NUTRITIONAL ASSESSMENT

Nutritional assessment in a pediatric intensive care unit (ICU) is almost similar to that done for adults. These include anthropometry, clinical, laboratory and review of previous and current intakes. Accurate assessment in terms of nutritional and metabolic parameters can go a long way in providing optimal nutritional support with a minimal number of complications.

In a critical child the most important anthropometric data is the weight and length or height. But given the conditions the child is in, one can obtain history of recent, involuntary weight loss (exceeding 5% within 1 month or 10% over 6 months). Of course, factors like fluid overload (in case of edema) may prevent the accurate determining of dry weight in the ICU.[1]

Physical examination should focus on signs of protein energy deficiency (such as temporal wasting), signs of specific micronutrient deficiency (such as anemia, glossitis or rash), hydration state and edema. Dry weight and height are used to calculate the ideal body weight, the percentage of ideal body weight and the basal metabolic index (BMI). If the onset of the illness is indolent, preadmission weight changes become easier to interpret. Obtaining a general idea of the patient's health status and nutrient intake helps determine the nutritional goals. Body status, edema, overall muscle bulk and evidence of pretemporal wasting should be assessed. Signs of depletion of muscle stores are indicative of preexisting malnutrition.

Serum albumin levels also help to identify malnourished patients and their risks for morbidity. This marker is considered a strong predictor of outcome of the disease status, but may be influenced by factors like protein synthesis, catabolism, renal losses and dilutional effects.

Balance studies also are used to assess the protein and energy requirements, like nitrogen (N) balance studies, which should be in the range of 2-4 g N/day (indicating an anabolic state). This may be difficult to achieve in a critically ill child, especially when hyperventilation is present.

Formulae using Harris Benedict equation or indirect calorimetry are often used for energy requirements. This equation is modified using correction factor adjustments which are easy to use, but the limitation of this study is the tendency to overestimate the caloric needs of a child in the ICU.[2]

Loss of body weight is a definitive accompaniment of protein energy malnutrition and provides a readily accessible indicator of altered nutritional status (>10% of ideal body weight indicating malnutrition), but as mentioned already, may not reflect the true status in presence of edema. Hepatic secretory proteins like albumin, transferrin, retinol binding protein and prealbumin are markers of visceral protein stores and used as methods of nutritional assessment, but are also influenced by other factors like disorders of hepatic function, protein losing states and acute infections or inflammation. Hence, these tests also may be of limited use in a child in the ICU.

Finally, in light of the above factors, consensus recommendations suggest that though there are multiple tests and combination of tests to assess nutritional status, no simple recommendation can be given regarding the 'best' test for assessing nutritional status. Use of any of these methods can be appropriate, providing the limitations are clearly understood. Although not studied in ICU patients, it is important to note that data in hospitalized patients suggest that clinical assessment of nutritional status, including weight loss (>10% of ideal body weight), is as reliable an indicator of malnutrition as more complex tests of nutritional assessment.[3]

INDICATIONS FOR NUTRITION SUPPORT IN THE ICU

It has been indicted that nutrition support for any critically ill patient is required where there is evidence of malnutrition or likelihood of development of malnutrition from inadequate oral intake because of a prolonged clinical course.[4]

In patients with respiratory failure, the presence or absence of mechanical ventilation is often the first cofactor in consideration of nutritional support. Mechanically, ventilated patients with respiratory failure also fall into one or two general categories—malnourished or hypermetabolic. However, if the respiratory failure is likely to be of short duration, aggressive nutritional support is not indicated.

Hypermetabolic patients, e.g. those with sepsis or acute respiratory distress syndrome (ARDS) are also fit candidates for nutritional support. The goal here is more to prevent further catabolism rather than repletion of nutritional status. The aim for nutritional support is mainly to minimize excessive protein losses, while at the same time provide maintenance substrates at levels that the body can deal with.

GENERAL GOALS AND PRINCIPLES

Goals of Nutritional Support

The general goals of nutritional support in the ICU patients are:

- To provide nutrients consistent with the patient's medical condition, nutritional status and available route of nutrient administration
- To prevent or treat macronutrient and micronutrient deficiencies
- To provide doses of nutrients compatible with existing metabolism
- To avoid complications related to the technique of dietary delivery
- To improve patient outcome such as those related to disease morbidity, e.g. body composition, tissue repair, organ function and those affecting medical mortalities and subsequent patient outcome.

Principles of Nutritional Support

Macronutrients (Calories and Protein Requirement)

In the critically ill patient, the goal of nutritional support is primarily maintenance rather than repletion. Aggressive nutrition support in order to bring the patient to a metabolic state from that of catabolic phase is not advisable, because by attempting to do so, complications, like increased carbon dioxide production, deposition of fat and glycogen in the liver and hyperglycemia may be encountered. Once the hypermetabolic phase is corrected, anabolism is favored and repletion occurs. During starvation, the body adapts to the decreased supply by decreasing its metabolic rate. Glycogen stores are first utilized within 24 hours and fat conserved till quite late in the process.

Carbohydrates and lipids should be so administered, so as to minimize lipolysis and protein degradation. Underfeeding and overfeeding both can be detrimental.[5] The hazards of overfeeding are well established:

1. Increased metabolic rate.
2. Increased oxygen consumption.
3. Hyperglycemia.
4. Dehydration secondary to osmotic diuresis.
5. Fatty liver.
6. Increased carbon dioxide production.
7. Ventilator dependency.
8. Immunosuppression.
9. Fluid overload.
10. Electrolyte imbalance.

For most patients administering 25 cals/ Kg/d appears to be adequate. These should be provided in a volume consistent with the total fluid needs of the patient which is generally 1 ml water/calorie. About 30 to 70 percent of the total calories administered can be given as glucose, i.e. up to 2-5 g glucose/Kg/d. The dose should be so adjusted as to maintain a blood glucose level >225 mg/dl, including regular insulin if required.[6]

Fats should comprise about 15 to 30 percent of the total calories administered per day. These should include omega 6 polyunsaturated fatty acids (PUFA), triglycerides in adequate dose, so as to prevent deficiency of essential fatty (EFA), i.e. about 5 to 7 percent of the total calories. Medium chain triglycerides (MCT) can also be used to provide calories.

Proteins should comprise about 1.5-2 g/Kg body weight/d. This works up to about 15 to 20 percent of the total calories. Patients are known to lose up to 1 percent of their body proteins per day. In hypermetabolic critically ill patients, protein degradation and synthesis typically increases but with a net protein decrease or catabolic effect.[7] However, it is recommended that the protein intake in any case should not exceed 1.8 g/Kg/d, except in severe losses and even then it can vary between 1.5-2.0 g/Kg/d.[8] Prolonged lack of protein support can cause nutritional deficiency.

The recommendations for an appropriate mix of carbohydrates and fats vary, but generally 60 to 70 percent carbohydrates are given with 20 to 30 percent fats.[9] The proportion is as follows:

Substrate Mix

Protein-----------------------------20% of the total calories (1-2 g/d)
Carbohydrates------------------60-70%
Fats---------------------------------20-30%

The role of certain amino acids like glutamine also has been stressed, as a semiessential amino acid. It serves as a major source of energy, being absorbed from the bowel lumen and is required for the rapidly dividing cells of the immune system.

The role of other essential semiessential amino acids contributing to multiple metabolic processes, like arginine and branched chain amino acids has been described but the benefit of their roles in the critically ill patient has failed to document any positive effects.[10]

Administering Nutrition

Having assessed the baseline nutritional status and requirements of a child in the ICU, the next step is to actually deliver the nutrients—when, how and what.

The optimal time to administer nutrition to an infant or child in an ICU may differ from one center to another. Assuming that the nutritional stores are already depleted, some authors have suggested initiating feeding in these children within a few days in infants, within 5 days in older children and within 7 days in adolescents.[11,12] Current data supports the initiation of enteral nutrition (EN) at the earliest possible after resuscitation. Small bowel feedings can usually be performed, even in the presence of gastric atony and colonic ileus. The role of agents formulated to improve gastric and intestinal motility is still controversial.

The presence of bowel sounds and the passage of flatus or stool are not necessary to initiate enteral feeds, especially when feedings are administered distal to the pylorus. However, any indication of abdominal distention might call for withholding of feeding and re-evaluation.

Nutrition support may be provided using either the enteral route (EN) or through the parenteral route (PN).

Enteral Nutrition

Oral feeding whenever feasible is the route of choice in any set up as it is the least invasive way of administering nutritional support in a functioning gut. Through this route, the gastrointestinal tract (GIT) is used and this helps to maintain the gut integrity and preserves the gut barrier function. The benefits of EN far outweigh those of PN:

1. It corrects the pH balance of the gut and helps reduce bacterial overgrowth. It is also known to reduce bacterial overgrowth.
2. It is known to reduce risk of gastrointestinal bleeding.
3. The gut motility also minimizes the delay in gastric emptying

In short, the accepted dictum is 'where the gut works, use it.' It has also been demonstrated that early EN (within 3 days of onset of illness on admission to ICU) is safe, efficient, cost-effective and associated with improved outcome.[13,14]

However, only when there is risk of high aspiration, should the decision of oral feeding be deferred. Small frequent feedings, as opposed to large bolus feeding should be the standard norm to be followed. In conditions when large volumes of feeds are not possible, the feeds may be concentrated to increase the caloric and protein density.

Secretory diarrhea may sometimes be encountered but this does not warrant cessation of enteral feeding, unless it exceeds 1000 ml/d. Generally, in the absence of any specific medical or surgical cause for the diarrhea, e.g. enterocolitis, antidiarrheal agents can help tide over the problem.

In conditions where the enteral route is not available in patients with respiratory failure who may not have a functioning GI tract, total parenteral nutrition (TPN) needs to be resorted to. The use of minimal EN feeding as 'trophic feeds' is also practiced by some experts along with TPN where possible.

Some of the conditions where oral route is inaccessible, and nasogastric (NG) feeding has to be resorted to are neurological disorders, inborn errors of metabolism like glycogen storage disease, cystic fibrosis, bronchopulmonary dysplasia, cerebral palsy and congenital heart diseases.

Certain complications are also known to be associated with enteral feedings like vomiting, diarrhea, abdominal distention and aspiration.

Enteral feedings are generally initiated as a continuous infusion pump with initial rate of 1-2 ml/Kg. body weight per hour. As the tolerance is built up, infusion rate is gradually increased every 6-8 hours. In case of NG feeding the general rule is to check the gastric residue. If found in excess of the previous hour's feeding, it is considered significant and hence the subsequent feed is withheld for an hour or two. If there is recurrent high gastric residue, use of prokinetics are indicated. In children who have been nil by mouth for longer periods, enteral feedings should be initiated very gradually.

Regular monitoring of the feeds for their electrolyte content as well as daily intake of calories, proteins and fluids should be monitored.

Parenteral Nutrition (PN)

When the nutritional route is inaccessible for any reason, over a fairly prolonged period parenteral nutrition is the alternative means of providing adequate nutrition. However, it may be kept in mind that PN is only the second line of choice and hence not without its own limitations. The debate over EN vs PN has been since the time PN was introduced, with no clear cut decisions yet as to which outweighs the other. It is observed that the choice of administering nutrition still largely depends upon case to case basis. Contraindications to enteral feeding include diffuse peritonitis, intestinal obstruction, intractable vomiting, paralytic ileus and severe prolonged diarrhea, hypotension and hemodynamic instability. Tables 18.1 and 18.2 give a comparative picture of the advantages and disadvantages of both EN and PN respectively. In such cases, total parenteral nutrition (TPN) plays an important role. Administration of 25 Kcals/Kg of expected body weight is adequate for most patients with normal BMI. In patients with lower BMI (<19), overfeeding is unlikely to result in refeeding syndrome which is manifested by electrolyte abnormalities, volume overload and congestive heart failure.[15] Therefore, gradually introducing TPN can ameliorate the risk of refeeding syndrome. To begin with 100-150 g dextrose and low concentration of sodium chloride can be administered with regular monitoring of electrolytes and blood sugars to achieve a state of euglycemia.

Overfeeding of carbohydrates results in respiratory quotient (RQ) close to 1.0, while fat based energy can yield an RQ close to 0.7 (mixed fuels, 0.8-0.9).[16]

The TPN composition has to be modified as per individual case to prevent refeeding in general especially carbohydrates. The protein requirement in TPN ranges from 1.2-1.5 g/Kg/d, which needs to be adjusted with periodic monitoring, to promote nitrogen (N) retention, and also support protein synthesis.[17]

Generally, observations in a critical care set up show that a positive N balance is rarely achieved due to the cytokine and catabolic hormone cascade preventing anabolism. There is not much risk of providing protein in higher amounts. In conditions where blood urea nitrogen (BUN) values exceed 100 mg/l, N intake might need to be decreased due to manifestation of symptoms of azotemia. In conditions of acute renal failure due to restriction of volume, the quality of feeding is limited in any case, but with chronic renal insufficiency, 0.8 g/Kg /d of protein is adequate. Similarly in conditions of hepatic encephalopathy, the protein content in the TPN might need to be reduced, but still the use of branched amino acids (BCCA) have shown good results.[18]

Table 18.1: Advantages and disadvantages of enteral nutrition

Advantages	*Disadvantages*
Physiologic	More time needed to reach full support
Preserves immune functions	Depends on functional status of GIT
Preserves gut barrier function	
Less costly than TPN	Multiple contraindications; intestinal obstruction
May blunt hypermetabolic response	Hemodynamic instability: high output enterocutaneous fistula, severe diarrhea

Table18.2: Advantages and disadvantages of parenteral nutrition

Advantages	*Disadvantages*
Available when enteral route contraindicated	Intestinal atropy
Can augment inadequate oral intake	Higher septic morbidity
Full support in less than 24 hours	
Contraindications are few	

The lipid component of TPN comprises omega 6 polyunsaturated fatty acids which are administered separately or as part of a 3-in-1 solution. The calories provided by fats up to 30 percent of total calories is considered safe especially when it is infused slowly as in the 3-in-1 solution. The main contraindication to lipids in TPN could be triglyceride levels >400 mg/l.

The remainder of the total calories can be provided as carbohydrates-between 3-5 g/Kg/d. The aim should be to maintain a blood glucose level <200mg/l and the dose can be adjusted accordingly. Mostly coinfusion of insulin is required on a sliding scale if indicated. Hyperglycemia >200 mg/l has been shown to be associated with nosocomial infections which can in fact nullify the benefit of nutritional support itself. TPN induced hyperglycemia may also be associated with severe stress (e.g. in postoperative patients) accompanied by rising plasma levels of counter regulatory hormones glucagon, epinephrine and cortisol.[17]

The fluid volume of TPN can be maintained at 1 l/day for patients of cardiac, pulmonary, postoperative and renal conditions in the ICU. This can provide approximately 1000 calories and 70 g of proteins which is usually adequate for the required feeding goal.

Vitamins and minerals are generally administered along with the TPN at the desired levels, along with any medications, e.g. histamine-2-receptor antagonists and metaclopramide.

In the pediatric ICU, PN is usually given as a continuous infusion, which makes it easier to manage the electrolytes, acid-base and fluid disturbances which may be generally encountered in this patient population.

MONITORING

There are no standard monitoring techniques for children on TPN, but electrolytes and glucose levels are usually done on a daily basis. Liver function tests may be monitored from time-to-time, due to the risk of vulnerability of this population to cholestatic liver disease.[19] Transition to EN is done as soon as the patient is able to tolerate it either orally or through the nasogastric route.

However, certain parameters may be checked to minimize complications and maximize the benefits of nutrition support, which may be summarized as follows:

1. Avoid overfeeding—a respiratory quotient of over 1 is indicative of overfeeding and may call for reduction of total calories (glucose and fat) to decrease carbon dioxide production.
2. Promote N retention and avoid protein overload.
3. Monitoring triglyceride clearance is recommended.
4. Adequate monitoring of fluid and electrolyte status is essential especially for potassium, phosphate, magnesium, calcium and zinc.
5. Periodic assessment of liver function tests.

Specialized Dietary Foods in the ICU

Besides the role of macro and micronutrients in the overall nutritional support of the ICU patient, a number of specific nutrients have evolved and their individual effects on specific metabolic functions are increasingly being recognized but the definitive role of each of them still remains to be defined clearly.[17]

Glutamine: It is an amino acid involved in a host of metabolic processes like during catabolic states, it is mobilized in increased amounts from peripheral tissues such as skeletal muscle. The outcome of administering glutamine in patients with catabolic states is still not clearly defined.

Branched chain amino acids (BCAAs): These are the essential amino acids (leucine, isoleucine and valine), crucial for protein synthesis. Given in dose of 0.5-1.2 g/Kg/d has demonstrated improved N retention with reduced urea genesis and increased protein synthetic functions.

Peptides in enteral formulations: These are proteins in their hydrolyzed forms and if added in enteral formulae may enhance enteral protein absorption.

Growth hormones: These are known to have a variety of metabolic effects like increased fat oxidation, increased rate of protein synthesis and improved immune responsiveness. Again their role in patient outcome is not defined.

Arginine: This is an amino acid having a role in a number of metabolic functions but its role in improving outcome in a patient in the ICU is yet unclear.

REFERENCES

1. Blackburn GL, Bristrain BR, Maini BS, et al. Nutritional and metabolic assessment of the hospitalized patient. JPEN, 1991;1:11-12.
2. Daly JM, Heymsfield SB, Head CA, et al. Human energy requirements. Overestimate by widely used prediction equation. Am J Clin Nutr 1985;42:11170-74 (Abstarct).
3. Thonnart N, Cuvelier B, Bracamonte M, et al. Metabolic utilization of LCT vs mixed MCT/LCT emulsion during IV infusion in man. Clin Nutr 1984; 4suppl):50-7.
4. Heyland DK. Nutritional support in the critically ill patient. Crit Care Clin. 1998;14:423-40.
5. Dabrowski GP, Rombeau JL. Practical critical nutritional management in the trauma ICU. Surg Clin North Am 2000;80:3.
6. Cerra FB, Benitez MR, Blackburn GL, Irwin RS, et al. Applied Nutrition in ICU Patients, ACCP Consensus Statement. Chest 1997;111:769-78.
7. Streat SJ, Hill GL. Nutrition in the management of critically ill surgical intensive care patients. World J Surg 1987;11:194-201.
8. Jolliet P, Pichard C, Biolo G, et al. ESCIM statement: Enteral nutrition in intensive care patients: A practical approach. Intensive Care Med 1998;24:848-59.
9. Pingleton SK. Nutrition in chronic critical illness. Clinics in Chest Medicine, March 2001; Vol 22, No.6.
10. Alexendar JW. Immunoenhancement via enteral nutrition. Arch Surg 1995;128:1242-5.
11. Norris KKG, Steinhorn DM. Nutritional management during critical illness in infants and children. Crit Care Med 1981;9:580-3.
12. Ford EG. Nutritional support of pediatric patients. Nutr Clin Prac 1996;11:183-91.
13. Adams S, Dellinger EP, Wertz MJ, et al. Enteral vs Parenteral nutritional support following laparatomy for trauma: A randomized perspective trial. J Trauma 1986; 10:882-91.
14. Kudsk KA, Croce MA, Fabian TC, et al. Enteral vs Parenteral feeding: Effects on septic morbidity after blunt and penetrating abdominal trauma. Ann Surg 1992; 215: 503-10.
15. Apovian CM Mc Mohan, MM, Bistrain BP. Guidelines for refeeding the marasmic patient. Crit Care Med 1990;18:1030-3.
16. Guenst JM, Nelson CD. Predictors of total parenteral nutrition induced lipogenesis. Chest 1994;105:553-9.
17. Cerra FB, Benitez MR, Blackburn GL, et al. Applied nutrition in ICU patients: A consensus statement of the American College of Chest Physicians. Chest 1997;111:769-78.

18. Fischer JE. Branched chain amino acid solutions in patients with liver failure: An early example of nutritional pharmacology. JPEN 14 (suppl):249S-56S.
19. Hofmann AF. Defective biliary secretion during total parenteral nutrition: Possible mechanisms and possible solutions. J Pediatr Gastroenterol 1995;20:376-90.

Chapter 19 Nutrition in Childhood Cancer

The most common type of childhood cancer known is acute lymphoblastic leukemia (ALL) and acute myeloblastic leukemia (AML). Leukemia accounts for 30 to 40 percent of all childhood cancers, lymphomas 9 to 15 percent and solid tumors like medulloblastoma, neuroblastomas, etc. for around 40 percent.

ALL is known to represent 80 percent of diagnoses followed by AML and the chronic subtypes of leukemia.[1]

Nutrition in such children is generally compromised due to various factors, some of which could be primary, i.e. the child may be undernourished from birth itself or may be born underweight or may subsequently get malnourished with progress of the disease. A recent study published in August 2004, issue of Cancer Causes and Control, researchers for the first time have linked the moth er's diet in her antenatal period to the onset of childhood leukemia. A systematic survey of 138 mothers, each having a child with ALL were interviewed regarding their detailed dietary history 12 months prior to pregnancy and the results were compared to age matched controls who did not have any child with cancer. Interestingly, it was seen that mothers who had higher intake of fruits and vegetables, and foods rich in proteins, had a lower risk of having a child with leukemia. According to the lead author of this study, fetal exposure to nutritional factors has a lot to do with what mothers eat. Within the fruit and vegetable groups, certain foods including carrots, string beans and cantaloupe stood out as having stronger links to lower childhood leukemia risk. It was also inferred that glutathione was the nutrient in the protein group with a strong link to lower cancer risk. Glutathione is an antioxidant found in both meat and legumes, and it plays an important role in the synthesis and repair of DNA as well as the detoxification of certain harmful compounds.[2]

It has also been shown that a consistently decreased risk of childhood leukemia with regular reported consumption of oranges/bananas and orange juice during the first 2 years of life.[3]

Consumption of common daily Chinese diet, like vegetables and soy foods may be associated with a reduced risk of childhood ALL, while consumption of cured/smoked meat/fish may increase the risk of childhood ALL.[4]

Breastfeeding for even a few months has been associated with decreased risk of childhood leukemia. An analysis of 14 studies conducted since 1988, found that overall, long-term breastfeeding was linked to 24 percent lower risk of ALL. Breastfeeding for 6 months or less appeared to lower risk of ALL by 12 percent. These observations based on International studies including more than 8,000 children with ALL or AML, offer a 'strong suggestion' that breastfeeding is protective as stated by Dr. Kwan of the University of California, Berkeley.[5]

RISK FACTORS FOR MALNUTRITION IN CHILDREN WITH CANCER

A number of disease associated factors contribute to risk of poor nutrition in these children, e.g. advanced stage solid tumors, ALL, multiple relapse leukemia and bone marrow transplantation. Cytokines like tumor necrosis factor (TNF), interleukin 1 and 6 and interferon also play an important role. A child with malignant disease has an increased energy expenditure, proteolysis and gluconeogenesis. The various risk factors in these children may be summed up as follows:

Decreased Food Intake: This could be due to:

- Unappetizing food, monotonous food, no variety
- Forced feeding
- Inadequate amounts of food
- Nausea, vomiting, sore mouth, diarrhea
- Repeated fasting for procedures from time to time
- Mucositis, swallowing or chewing difficulties.

Increased Nutrient Requirements: These are increased in children with cancer due to:

- Metabolic stress /impact of the illness itself
- Wound or fistula losses.

Decreased Absorption: Despite adequate intake, most children might not be absorbing the nutrients optimally due to:

- Disease or treatment involved like chemotherapy
- Enteropathy or pancreatic exocrine impairment
- Infections due to suppressed immunity in these children.

Goals of Nutritional Support in Children with Cancer

- To help achieve normal growth and weight gain
- To continue normal activities
- To reduce morbidity and minimize complications
- To maximize quality of life

Management

To initiate any nutritional intervention in a child, the first step is to establish a base line nutritional status. This is done by assessing the nutritional of the child which involves.

- ***Anthropometry:*** This involves weight, height, mid arm circumference.
- ***SGA*:** This tool is known to be more sensitive as compared to weight or height which may vary with various factors, e.g. large tumors.
- ***Dietary intake:*** This can be done by 24 hours recall and food frequency questionnaire.

Nutritional Requirements

Calories: The energy needs are increased in such patients due to increased metabolic needs. This will help in ensuring normal growth and development as well as prevent increased losses. Some of the ways how energy of the food can be increased are:

- Use of butter, cream, etc. into the foods offered
- Use of skim milk powder to the milk or any food offered. This will increase the density of the food without increasing the volume
- Use of sweetened condensed milk.

Proteins: The child normally requires adequate proteins for his growth and body building. However, in patients with cancers, these requirements are further enhanced for growth and tissue repair. Proteins may be increased by

- Use of skim milk powder which is concentrated milk powder, in preparations, milk, custard, ice cream, etc.
- Use of eggs or cheese may be incorporated in any form as desired by the child.

Minerals and vitamins: These are equally important for adequate absorption and maintenance of body functions. Fat soluble vitamins like A, D and E serve as antioxidants, which help build immunity in the child and prevent from recurring infections. Fruits and green vegetables are good sources for these. However, care should be taken to avoid raw vegetables or partially cooked food due to the risk of contamination due to microbial growth. Soft cheese, fish and mushrooms are better avoided due to fear of contamination. These precautions are required for neutropenic children.

Feeding a Fussy Child

As cautioned earlier, children with leukemia or any cancer tend to be quite difficult to feed optimally. The reasons may be varied which are elaborated in the beginning of this chapter. Some basic guidelines for encouraging a 'poor eater' are:

1. Small frequent feeds should be offered, distributed over the day – 3 main meals and 3 in between snacks.
2. Powder packing of food by increasing the density of the food, e.g. addition of butter, cheese, cream to sauces or foods. A dish may be fried instead of boiled or baked.
3. Variety should be added in the diet.
4. Nutritional supplements may be added to beverages offered to them.
5. Flexibility of meal timings, parentral involvement and menu choices should be considered individually.
6. Group eating in the ward may encourage healthy eating.
7. Addition of sauces to gravies can improve flavors and palatability of food besides increasing moisture which helps swallowing, if the mouth is dry.
8. Often a child is totally unable to eat during the course of chemotherapy, but may accept adequately during the in-between cycles. In such cases, it could be helpful if he/she is made to eat during the 'off chemotherapy days' and the deficit be compensated during these periods.

ENTERAL FEEDING AND PARENTERAL NUTRITION

When adequate feeding is compromised over an extended period in children with cancer, enteral tube feeding is an alternative option. Most children are anorexia and just not able to ingest enough to be able to meet the optimal requirements. If left in such condition without feeding, there is risk of severe malnutrition with growth faltering. Therefore, it is recommended that enteral tube feed or parenteral nutrition may be resorted to if:[6]

- The child is malnourished at diagnosis
- Loss of >5% body weight
- Weight for height <90 percent
- Drop in across two centiles
- Food intake <80 percent estimated requirement
- Bone marrow transplantation patient.

Special blenderised feeds can be easily prepared to be fed by the enteral route. Milk based formulation enriched with skim milk powder, eggs, fats, etc. can be tailor made to suit an individual child to meet the nutrient requirements. Since, quite a few of such children requiring tube feeding are also able to take orally, though not adequately, it would be a good idea to encourage the child to eat as much as possible during the day and the deficit can be compensated by tube feeding at night or during the day, depending upon the volume required to be fed. However, in a few number of cases nasogastric tube may be difficult to insert due to mucositis or vomiting. In such cases parenteral route for providing nutrition may be considered. In conditions of severe gastrointestinal complications due to chemotherapy, enteral route may be difficult to provide, in which case parenteral nutrition can be resorted to. Some of the common problems associated with enteral nutrition are diarrhea, vomiting, regurgitation or aspiration.

One of the nutritional complications in these children is gain in weight leading to overweight/obesity. This is due to reduced physical activity during the course of treatment. Almost 4 percent of children being treated for ALL have been found to be obese.[6] Reduced physical activity may also result in reduction in bone mineral density consequent to decreased activity, reduced calcium intake and the effects of corticosteroid treatment.[5]

REFERENCES

1. Ries LAGSM, Gurney JG, Tamira T, et al. Cancer incidence and survival among children and adolescents. United States SEER Program 1976-95, National Cancer Institute, SEER program NIH Pub Bethesda, MD, 1999, pp 17-34.
2. Jensen C. New study suggests link between maternal diet and childhood leukemia risk. Science Daily. 2004;24.
3. Marilyn l Kwan, Gladys Block, Steve Selvin, Stacy Month and Patricia A Buffer. Food consumption by children and the risk of childhood acute leukemia. Am J Epidemiology, Vol 160, No. 11, pp 1098-1107.
4. Reuters Health. wwwreutershealth.com.
5. Koletzko B. Karger, John WL Puntis. Nutritional challenges in special conditions and diseases, Hemato Oncology In: Pediatric Nutrition in Practice, Ed. 2008, pp 244-47.
6. Oeffinger KC, Mertens AC, Sklar CA, et al. Obesity in adult survivors of childhood acute lympoblastic leukemia: a report from the Childhood Cancer Survivor Study. J Clin Oncol 2003;21:1359-65.

Chapter 20 Nutrition Support in Children with HIV/AIDS

Acquired immunodeficiency syndrome (AIDS) is a serious condition comprising a deficiency of the immune system and other complex and severe diseases, leading to death. It is the final stage in progression of diseases resulting from human immunodeficient virus infection (HIV+) which can be transmitted to other persons.[1]

The disease was first identified in 1980s around Africa and identified as 'slim' disease since the affected patients looked very lean and was later named as AIDS in 1982 and in 1986, reported to be an HIV infection.[2] The number of people living with HIV increased 3-4 times from 1990-2008 and is still rising. Young people (15-24 years old) account for half of all new HIV infections worldwide and about 6,000 become infected with HIV everyday.[1]

Infants born to mothers who are HIV+ are generally of low birth weight related to low gestational age, having high viral loads.[3]

PATHOPHYSIOLOGY

AIDS is caused by the human immunodeficiency virus (HIV-1). HIV enters the cell and after replication, induces cell dysfunction or death. Cells of the immune system are the most commonly affected.

The lymphocytes which are part of the immune system are of two types–B cells, responsible for humoral immunity and T cells, responsible for cell mediated immunity.

The T cells are either helper (CD4+) or suppressor (CD 8+). CD4 cells enhance the operation of the entire immune system, while the CD8 cells shut down the immune response after the foreign antigens have been destroyed. In healthy individuals, the numbers of helper cells (CD4) are twice as the CD8 cells, where as in patients with AIDS, it is vice versa, i.e. the CD4 counts are suppressed drastically.[4]

Breastfeeding is one of the most common and easy routes of transmission of the disease from HIV infected mothers to their infants. The rate of the infection in babies is cumulative and roughly constant throughout the breastfeeding periods.

There are a number of factors, which influence the rate of transmission from mother to child, while breastfeeding. These are maternal clinical immunologic status, plasma and breast milk viral load and condition of the breast (e.g. mastitis, cracked nipples, etc.).

EFFECT OF HIV ON NUTRITION

Nutrition plays an important role in HIV affected mothers and their infants. Poor nutrition is commonly seen in such mothers and malnutrition can play an important role in the progression of the disease. In children HIV infection can result in failure to thrive, stunting and wasting. There is poor feeding, malabsorption, tissue catabolism and psycho social factors. Figure 20.1 highlights the effects of HIV on the nutritional status of the children. Higher viral load can further accelerate growth failure. Infected children born to HIV+ mothers have early stunting which is sustained, and are malnourished but not necessarily wasted.[5] It has been postulated that HIV does not affect the birth weight of the child, but significant postnatal growth abnormalities even in the asymptomatic child can occur rapidly.[6] The impairment of growth is generally observed by 2 years of age, while some have also reported such deficits as early as 4 months also in some infected infants.[7,8] Children with HIV, manifest preferential loss of lean body mass as compared to fat mass, which may or may not be associated with weight loss.[6]

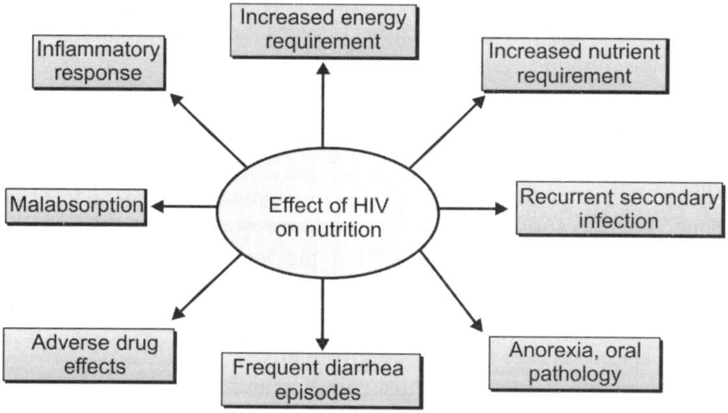

Fig. 20.1: Effect of HIV on nutrition

CAUSES OF MALNUTRITION IN HIV INFECTED CHILDREN

The main obvious cause of failure to gain weight is attributed to increased expenditure. They tend to burn 10 percent more calories while resting, compared to those who are in infected. Besides this decreased energy intake is an added contributory factor. This could be aggravated by associated anorexia and inability to eat. Conditions like oral thrush, diarrhea, nausea and vomiting may all be linked to decreased intake by these patients. Malabsorption of the GIT of all the nutrients, especially fat from food is another significant causative factor of decreased intake.

OXIDATIVE STRESS IN HIV+/AIDS PATIENTS

Children with HIV+ infection may have decreased levels of antioxidants like vitamins, sulfhydryl (SH) potential and total glutathione (GSH). Malnutrition and diarrhea can also cause a decrease in the levels of vitamins and SH compounds.

AIDS progression can also be caused by some toxic foods and drinks and certain toxic chemicals, herbicides, alcohol and tobacco.

Studies have demonstrated significantly decreased blood levels of vitamin A, beta carotene, vitamin E and the antioxidative status in HIV+/AIDS patients, as compared to healthy individuals. This is mainly as a result of poor nutrition with lowered dietary antioxidants.

IMMUNITY AND OTHER CO-FACTORS IN AIDS

Even if people are infected with HIV, they may remain asymptomatic for a long duration, but their immune system gradually becomes weak till the symptoms appear. The immune system in these patients is severely affected, thereby exposing them to increased susceptibility to opportunistic infections, which are unlikely in healthy individuals. Common symptoms are fever, chills, sweats, lymphadenopathy, weakness and weight loss. They are prone to be infected by harmful infectious microorganisms like bacteria, viruses, fungi and parasites. These opportunistic infections accentuate malnutrition and wasting syndromes.

ROLE OF NUTRITION IN HIV+/AIDS CHILDREN

Nutrition interventions have a wide range of benefits for HIV related outcomes.[9] The goal of nutrition support in HIV+/AIDS patients should be:

- Promote optimal growth
- Lean tissue repletion (prevent malnutrition)

- Enhance quality of life by providing adequate calories and nutrients
- Improve immunity (increase in CD4 count) by improving intake.

NUTRITIONAL REQUIREMENTS FOR HIV INFECTED CHILD

Energy

HIV infection affects nutrition through increases in resting energy expenditure, reductions in food intake nutrient malabsorption and loss and complex metabolic alterations, leading to weight loss and wasting in AIDS. There is need to increase energy intake by at least 10 percent of the recommended dietary intake (RDA) in asymptomatic HIV infected children to maintain growth. But if there is already significant weight loss and the patient is symptomatic, an increase of 50 to 100 percent energy above the RDA for healthy children is recommended.[10]

An oral intake of a wide variety of nutrient dense foods combined with oral supplementation and nutritional counseling should help to meet the increased needs. A high fat supplement or recipe which includes high amounts of oil, cream or butter can help meet the increased demands.

In children unable to accept orally, as per required amounts, nasogastric feeding should be considered. This can be done in addition to a free oral intake during the day, as a night time regimen. Commercial supplements can be helpful in supplementing the oral intake if the child is unable to consume adequately. Parenteral nutrition should be reserved for HIV infected children, who continue to lose weight on an aggressive enteral program, or for children who have persistent diarrhea with weight loss or severe recurrent or chronic pancreatic or biliary tract disease.

Protein

There is not much data available to support increase in protein requirements over and above the RDA (12-15% of total energy intake). However, with an increase in the total energy, the intake of protein is also proportionately increased.

Micronutrients

Due to the decreased intake by children with HIV/AIDS infected children, deficiency of micronutrients are bound to occur. This may further accelerate progression of HIV disease leading to worsened nutritional status.[10] Nutritional supplement may also restore intestinal absorption and increase CD4 count in affected children. As per WHO recommendations, children younger than 5 years born to HIV infected mothers, living in resource limited settings should be supplemented periodically (4-6 months) with vitamin A in doses as per healthy children.[10] Suggested vitamin A doses are 1 lac IU for children 6-12 months and 2 lac IU for children above 1 year.

Various workers have proposed high and specific doses of vitamins (A, B_1, B_2 and folic acid, C, D and E) for children with HIV/AIDS infection.

Vitamin A and β-carotene are considered to have a role in maintaining and protecting skin and epithelium and increasing immune functions.[11]

Vitamins B complex functions as co-enzymes for energy metabolism and increase in lean body mass.[12,13]

Vitamins C and E exert an antioxidant role and act in preventing oxidative stress, while minerals like iron, selenium and zinc are known to act as co-factors for antioxidant enzymes.[14]

Affect of Antiretroviral Therapy (ARVT)

The nutritional status of individuals put on highly active antiretroviral therapy (HAART) is known to improve, independent of its effects, suppression and immune status, although wasting can still be seen in some patients.[15] The first beneficial effect to be noticed after beginning of HAART, are gains in arm and muscle circumference. The improvement is seen maximum in children with lowest base line BMI and who have more advanced HIV disease.

ARVT is also known to cause severe nausea and vomiting which can decrease the intake of the child. Besides, there are other metabolic complications like derangement in glucose metabolism, bone metabolism and lactic academia, associated with initial treatment of ARV drugs. Like in adults, children are also affected by the metabolic effects of HAART and have a significant risk of lipodystrophy.

Feeding of the HIV Exposed Infant

Infants on breastfeeds are also at risk through breastfeeding. The risk of HIV transmission through breastfeeding is directly related to the health, viral load and immune status of the mother. Infection occurs at an average rate of about 8.9 HIV transmissions per 100 child years of breastfeeding.[16]

HIV positive mothers are recommended to avoid breastfeeding if replacement feeding is affordable, feasible, sustainable and safe (AFASS).[17] Very often in poor socioeconomic strata, mothers tend to initiate breastfeeding. WHO recommends exclusive breastfeeding for these mothers and also early cessation of feeding. Infants who are not breastfed or who stop breastfeeding early and do not have access to safe and nutritious replacement foods are at increased risk of malnutrition, diarrhea and other illness and death.[18]

WHO/UNICEF/UNAIDS/UNPFA[19] has framed certain guidelines which can help in deciding which feeding option would best suit an individual HIV infected mother depending upon various social and environmental factors. These are summarized in Table 20.1.

Table 20.1: Considerations for deciding on the most feasible option for HIV+ mothers

	Most feasible option		*Replacement feeding or expressed, heat-treated breast milk*
	Breastfeeding/ wet-nursing	*Unclear*	
Drinking-water supply	River, stream, pond, or well	Public standpipe	Piped water at home or ability to purchase clean water
Latrine	None or pit latrine	VIP latrine	Waterborne latrine
Income	Less than USD 15 available for formula each month	USD 15 available for formula most months	USD 15 available for formula every month (unless using expressed breast milk)
Food storage	No refrigerator or regular electricity supply available	Access to refrigerator with regular electricity supply, but not at home	Refrigerator at home with regular electricity supply
Preparation and fuel	Inability to boil water and utensils for every feed	Ability to boil water for every feed but with effort	Ability to boil water for every feed
Ability to prepare night feeds	Preparation of replacement feeds at night difficult	Preparation of replacement feeds at night possible but with effort	Preparation of replacement feeds at night possible
Family and community support	Breastfeeding expected, and family unaware of HIV status	Replacement feeding acceptable, but family unaware of HIV status; or breastfeeding expected, but family aware of HIV status and willing to help with feeding	Family aware of HIV status and willing to help with feeding

Ref. WHO, UNICEF, UNAIDS, UNFPA[20]

WHO/UNAIDS/UNICEF[20] recommends several variations of exclusive breast feeding and replacement milk for infants of HIV infected mothers (Table 20.2).

Table 20.2: WHO/UNAIDS/UNICEF feeding options for infants on HIV infected mothers

Breast milk	*Replacement milk*
Exclusive breastfeeding by the mother for 6 months and continuing till age of 2 years or as long as mothers choose.	Commercial infant formula prepared as per manufacturer's directions
Exclusive breastfeeding by the mother with early cessation, with rapid weaning to replacement milk as early as feasible.	Fresh full cream milk; with added water, sugar and micronutrients, boiled before use.
Breast milk expression with heat treatment; expressed milk fed by cup.	Evaporated full cream milk or powdered full cream milk; with added water, sugar and micronutrients.
Wet nursing by an HIV uninfected mother.	

All feeding options recommend introduction of complementary foods at 6 months of age.
Refer.[19] WHO/UNAIDS/UNICEF (2000)

Breastfeeding

Mothers who do breastfeed due to conditions mentioned earlier need to exercise some preventive measures so as to minimize the risk of transmission through breast milk which can be summed up as follows:

1. Practice exclusive breastfeeding ideally for 6 months.
2. Stop breastfeeding as soon as replacement feeding is acceptable. Feasible, affordable, sustainable and safe-preferably not later than 6 months.
3. Good lactation management (early initiation, attachment, positioning, frequent feeding, learning to express) can prevent breastfeeding problems like cracked nipples, engorgement and mastitis.
4. When cracked or bleeding nipples, mastitis or abscesses do occur, continue feeding from the unaffected side, and regularly express from the affected side and discard.
5. Oral thrush or mouth ulcers in the infant should be promptly treated.
6. Expressed milk can be heat treated in conditions during periods of increased risk of transmission, secondary to cracked nipples or during transmission from exclusive breastfeeding to replacement feeding.
7. Condoms should be used by sexually active mothers throughout the lactation period.

Replacement Feeding

Replacement feeding is given as a substitute for breastfeeding, in the form of formula milk before 6 months. After 6 months, this feeding is continued but with introduction of semi solid food. This is especially important for mothers diagnosed recently with HIV infection or progressed to AIDS (or whose CD4 count is less than 200/μl) who should offer replacement feeding to prevent high risk of transmission to the infant. Most commercial infant formulae are appropriate if prepared hygienically and as per directions on the packing. Infants who also test positive for HIV infection can be offered breastfeeding by mothers testing positive for HIV, since preventing breastfeeding for them will not make any difference. It would be advisable for such mothers to continue on exclusive breastfeeding for 6 months, but beyond that complementary feeding should be started in any case, in the form of juice, rice, potatoes, dark green vegetables, etc.

Mothers who wean from exclusive breastfeeding to replacement feeding need to consider some important factors for smooth transition:

1. Infants should be allowed a period of 2 days to 2 weeks to adjust to the new feeding pattern.
2. The infant should be acclimatized to the use of cup feeding by using expressed breast milk (EBM).
3. Breastfeeding can be eliminated for one cup feed and EBM can be replaced in the cup.
4. EBM should be discarded if nipples are sore, cracked or engorged. Cold compresses can help mitigate inflammation due to engorgement.
5. Once cup feeding has begun and accepted by the infant, reintroduction of breastfeeds should be avoided, nor should breastfeeding be used to pacify the child.
6. In case EBM has to be given, it should be heat treated and given by cup.

At 6 months, if it is still not conducive to 'AFASS', continuation of breastfeeding is recommended along with complementary foods. EBM of HIV+ mothers, if adequately heat treated, will not transmit HIV infection and nutritionally and immunologically safe. This can also be done in conditions when there is increased risk of transmission through cracked nipples. Wet nursing is a good option for feeding infants, in communities where it is acceptable and feasible, but care should be taken that they be tested before and after 6 weeks of starting.

REFERENCES

1. http://www.who.int (WHO and FAO)
2. http://www.aids.org (How many people have HIV and AIDS? AID. ORG, Inc-A-A project of Community Partners, 2007).
3. Katz A. The evolving art of caring for pregnant women with HIV infection. J Obstet Gynecol Neonatal Nurs 2003;32:102-08.
4. Samour PQ, Helm KK and Lang CE, Olsen LG, Cutroni R and Furuta L. Pediatric Acquired Immunodeficiency Syndrome. In: Handbook of Pedutric Nutrition 2nd ed. 2004, Publishers Joes and Barlette, pp 453-63.
5. Bobat R, Coovdia H, Moodley D, Coutsoudis A, Gouws E. Ann Trop Pediatr 201;21(3):203-10.
6. Miller TL. Nutritional aspects of pediatric HIV infection. In: Walker WA, Watkins JB Eds. Nutrition in Pediatrics. 2nd ed. Hamilton, Ontario; C Decker; 1996: 534-50.
7. Miller TL, Evaas S, Orav EJ, Morris V, et al. Growth and body composition in children with human immunodeficiency virus-1. Am J Clin Nutr. 1993;57:588-92.
8. McKinney RE, Robertson JR. Effect of human immunodeficiency virus infection on the growth of young children. Duke Pediatric AIDS Clinical Trials Unit. J Pediatr. 1993;123:579-82.
9. Baruchal S, Wainberg MA. The role of oxidative stress in disease progression in individuals infected by the human immunodeficient virus. J Leukoc Biol 1992;52:111-4.
10. WHO: Requirements for People Living with HIV/AIDS: Report of a Technical Consultation. Geneva, WHO, 2003.
11. Falio FN, Helio V, Alceu A, et al. Recommended dose for repair of serum vitamin A levels in patients with HIV infection/AIDS may be insufficient because of high urinary losses. Nutrition 2006;22:483-9.
12. Davidhizae R and Dunn C. Nutrition, and the client with AIDS. J Pract Nurs 1998;48:16-25; quiz 26-8.
13. Lands L. A comprehensive approach to HIV: The synergism of complementary therapies combined with aggressive medical management. Carl Vogel Foundation, Washington DC 1992.
14. Chandra RK. Nutrition and the immune system: An introduction. Am J Clin Nutr 1997:19:460 S.
15. Rousseau MC, Molines C, Moreau J, Delmont J. Influence of highly active anti retroviral therapy on micronutrients profiles of HIV infected patients. Ann Nutr Metab 200, 44 (56): 212-16.
16. The breastfeeding and HIV International Transmission Study (BHITS Group. Late postnatal transmission of HIV-1 in breastfed children: an individual patient data meta-analysis.

17. WHO. New Data on the prevention of Mother to child transmission of HIV and their Policy Implications: Conclusions and recommendations. Geneva, 11-13 Oct. 2000.
18. WHO Collaborative Team on the role of breastfeeding in the prevention of Infant mortality. Effect of breastfeeding on infant and child mortality due to infectious diseases in less developed countries. A pooled analysis. Lancet, 2000;353:451-55.
19. WHO, UNICEF, UNAIDS, UNPFA: HIV and Infant Feeding: A guide for Health Care Managers and Supervisors. Geneva, WHO, 2003.
20. WHO, UNAIDS, UNICEF: HIV and Infant Feeding Counseling: A Training Course, Geneva, WHO/UNAIDS/UNICEF, 2000. WHO document WHO/FCH/CAH/00. 2-4.

Chapter 21

Diet in Dental Health

Dental health in children in terms of nutrition is still not widely recognized by parents, nor has it been emphasized upon by the community. In fact, diet plays an important role in dental health especially after the eruption of teeth. It is only after the age of 3-4 years when teeth have erupted completely, or till ages 6-7 years when a child is brought to a pedodontist for any dental problems.[1] Now with increasing awareness of parents regarding the dental health of their children, they tend to bring them for examination as soon as any kind of abnormality or problem is detected. But before that period, the fact is generally ignored that a good diet and healthy eating practices can actually defer their visit to the pedodontist for any dental problem. It is here that the role of the pediatrician along with the dietician comes-that of educating the parents regarding good dental health and the influence of the child's feeding behavior (right from infancy onwards) upon dental health of the child. Nutrition affects the teeth during development and malnutrition may exacerbate periodontal and oral infectious diseases.[2, 3]

TOOTH DEVELOPMENT AND STRUCTURE

There are two sets of teeth which appear in one's lifetime. First is the primary set or the 'milk teeth' as they are known, which appear from age of 6 months onwards and the second one- the permanent set which gradually replaces the primary set between the ages of 6-12 years. The primary set comprises 20 teeth, while the permanent set comprises 32 teeth. The tooth consists of 3 types tissues (Fig. 21.1):

Enamel: This is a hard substance which forms the outer surface of the tooth and is composed of calcium and phosphate. This is the only part exposed to the oral environment.

Dentin: It is the major component of the tooth which is supplied with nerves and blood vessels.

Cementum: The dentin is covered by a thin layer of bone like material which forms the cementum. This holds the teeth in the jaw.

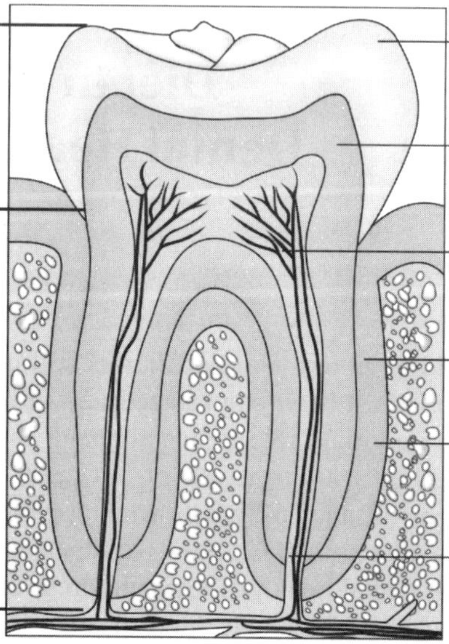

Fig. 21.1: Structure of a tooth

The mineralization of the teeth begins before birth, with the process of enamel formation being completed during the first year of life. It is at this stage of infancy when the feeding pattern of the child can be influenced (e.g. fluoride in the water, bottle feeding or bottle caries), although diet can continue to influence the teeth after eruption through local effects.

NUTRITIONAL INFLUENCE ON THE PRE-ERUPTED TEETH

The teeth begin to develop at 6-8 weeks in vitro and continue to be influenced by systemic nutrition till they erupt. They go through 3 main stages of development before erupting into the oral cavity:

Proliferative stage: This is the initial stage when there is hyperplastic growth of the teeth, and requires adequate proteins for the process. Vitamins A and C are essential for the enamel forming cells (ameloblasts) and dentin forming cells (odontoblasts).

Matrix formation stage: The matrix is mainly collagen and for this vitamin C and adequate amounts of protein is required from infancy itself. Deficiency of these nutrients can lead to susceptibility to caries and altered or malformed teeth.

Pre-eruptive stage: This is a process of teeth maturation and hardening to increase the resistance of enamel to dental caries. Excessive sugar intake during the pre-eruptive stage can adversely affect the maturation process.

ROLE OF SPECIFIC NUTRIENTS ON TOOTH MATURATION

During the process of matrix formation liberal calcification of the ameloblasts and the odontoblasts occurs, forming a calcified mass of tricalcium phosphate. This calls for a good source of calcium, phosphate and vitamin D for adequate mineralization. If during the first 6-8 years of life any portion of these ameloblasts are injured or killed due to deficiency of vitamin D, high fever or administration of antibiotics like tetracyclines, enamel discoloration and disfigurement can result. It has been suggested that the most critical age is 10 months and between 2 and a half to 5 years, when the enamel cells are most sensitive to any stress.[4]

DEMINERALIZATION AND REMINERALIZATION—ROLE OF FLUORIDE

When there is inadequate brushing or cleaning of the teeth, a sticky substance called plaque develops. This plaque bacterium produces acids by fermentation of sugars, decreasing the pH at the tooth surface. The sugars may be already present in the foods or produced by starch breakdown in the mouth. These acids dissolve the minerals in the enamel (calcium and phosphorus), a process which is known as demineralization. Enamel demineraliztaion takes place below a pH of about 5.5, which is called the 'critical pH'.

The acids produced in the mouth are gradually neutralized by saliva. This causes the pH of the tooth surface to rise above the critical pH. The increase in pH causes a return of the dissolved calcium and phosphate back to the enamel. This is called 'remineralization'.

In the event of constant eating during the daytime, chance of remineralization is greatly reduced. A gap of 2-3 hours between 2 meals can spare the damage done by demineralization and gives time for the teeth to repair themselves.[5]

Fluoride is an important nutrient required for mineralization of the tooth, and an adequate amount of it in the diet or water during the preeruptive stage can ensure good teeth which can be caries resistant. The tooth enamel is known to become fully mineralized during the preeruptive maturation period and it is during this phase that a significant amount of fluoride is acquired. Out of the 1 mm (1,000 µm) thickness of the tooth enamel, only the outer 30-50 µm of the enamel surface acquires significant amount of fluoride.[6] Fluoride deposition continues in the external enamel surface during the late pre-eruptive period, well after calcification is complete. The higher the concentration of fluoride in the outer layers of the surface enamel, the more caries resistant is the tooth.

Fluoride is known to protect the teeth against dental caries. It can be incorporated into the teeth during formation. It can also act locally once the tooth has erupted making the enamel surface of the tooth more resistant to acid and it also reduces the production of acids by bacteria in the mouth, thereby increasing the remineralization process.

DENTAL CARIES

Dental caries is the progressive destruction of the teeth by acid produced by the bacteria on the tooth surface. This happens over a period of time when the process of demineralization exceeds that of remineralization. Dental caries is widely prevalent and is increasing in some developing countries undergoing nutritional transition.[7]

Epidemiological studies have demonstrated evidence between the amount and frequency of free sugars intake and dental caries. Other carbohydrates especially cooked starch, e.g. in crisps, which can be broken down by enzymes in saliva to component sugars, may also damage the teeth although to a lesser degree.

Sucrose is most commonly associated with caries, although glucose, fructose and maltose seem equally cariogenic. The amount of sugar consumed at one time is less important than how often sugar containing foods are consumed. The longer the teeth are exposed to sugary foods, greater is the time during which the tooth are exposed to low pH levels inducing demineralization. The sugars present in complex forms or in combination with other foods, can reduce the impact of damage on the teeth, thus reducing the risk of caries, since other foods hinder the drop in pH.

Fruit juice compared to fruits can be more cariogenic. The explanation lies in the fact that sugars in fruits are held in cells of the fruit and are not released until chewing breaks down the cells. On the contrary, in fruit juice, sugars are no longer held in the cells of the fruit, thus causing development of caries. This can be aggravated more in children in whom the teeth are exposed for a longer time, e.g. in a feeding bottle.

The sticky nature of carbohydrates also tends to promote risk of caries, since foods like dry fruits or chocolates or certain sweets can stick to the mouth, thus reducing the pH in the mouth for a long time, leading to demineralization.

A common example of the effect of protracted exposure of teeth to sugar is the so called 'nursing bottle syndrome' leading to 'bottle caries'.[8,9] This is characterized by extensive and rapid loss of tooth surface in all the upper teeth including the lower molars. This is commonly prevalent in the 2-4 years old children who continue to nurse the bottle as a pacifier at bed time. The bottle is not only used for milk, but also for other beverages like tea, juices or sweetened water. The beverage tends to accumulate around the upper teeth. The interaction between the sugars and the teeth lowers the pH, encouraging demineralization, which decalcifies and destroys the teeth. During the child is asleep, lack of adequate salivary flow leads to stagnation of fermenting beverage and neutralizes its acids. This results in painful and broken down carious teeth.[7] It is therefore recommended that mothers be educated regarding measures to keep in mind while feeding their children which are:

Try to avoid use of feeding bottles, especially as pacifiers at bed time

- In situations where a child has become emotionally dependent upon the bottle, plain water should be used which can gradually dissuade him away from the bottle.
- The plaque must be removed before offering the next feed by brushing or wiping it away with a gauze pad.

DENTAL EROSION

Dental erosion differs from dental caries, since the former is not caused by bacteria but by action of acid, which could be either gastric or foods and drinks. Erosion can also occur in children with gastroesophageal reflux where there is a recurrent problem of vomiting or regurgitation. The erosion of the enamel and the dentin from the tooth can cause exposure of the pulp leading to pain and sensitivity to hot or cold foods.[10]

Some of the common foods and drinks consumed by children like soft drinks, fruit juices or carbonated fizz drinks and vinegar based foods all are acidic to some degree and can contribute to dental erosion. Children between 5-14 years are most prone to dental erosion due to their increased tendency to rely on such foods.[11]

Prevention of Dental Caries

Avoidance of acidic foods and drinks is the only prevention for dental erosion. Moreover, the duration of contact the teeth are exposed to the acidic food or beverage also determines the degree of erosion the teeth undergo. Using a straw for beverages can help minimize the risk and duration of exposure the teeth are subjected to. Swishing drinks or fruit juice in the mouth as most children playfully do should be avoided. Secondly, after consuming such foods and beverages, the teeth should not be brushed for at least one hour, since immediate brushing (e.g. at bed time just after dinner), will prevent the remineralization of the enamel to take place.

REFERENCES

1. Nizel AE. Nutritional support for optimizing children's dental health. In: Textbook of Pediatric Nutrition (Ed). Suskind RM. Raven Press 1981;583-95.
2. Infente PF, Gillespie GM. Enamel hypoplasia in relation to caries in Guatemalan children. J Dent Res 1977;56:493-8.
3. Infente PF, Owen GM, Russel AL. Dental caries in preschool Apache Indian children. J Dent Res 1977;54:915.
4. Massler M and Schour I. Am j Orthod Oral Surg 1946;32:495-517.
5. British Nutrition Foundation. Dental Health, 2004.
6. Melberg JR. Fluoride in preventive dentistry. J Prev Dent. 1977; 4:8-20.
7. Moynihan P, Peterson PE. Diet, Nutrition and the prevention of dental diseases. Public Health Nutr 2004;7 (1A): 201-26.
8. Bernick S. What the pediatrician should know about children's teeth IV. Baby-Bottle syndrome. Clin Pediatr 1971;10: 243-4.
9. Castano F. Penn Dent J 1972;39:8-11
10. Gandara BK, Truelove EL. Diagnosis and management of dental erosion. The J of Contemporary Dental Practice. 1999, Vol. 1, No. 1 Nov. 15.
11. Dugmoro CR, Rock WP. A multifactorial analysis of factors associated with dental erosion. Brit Dent J 2004;196(5):283-6.

Index

D

E